How Can I Tell You?

Secrecy and Disclosure with Children When a Family Member Has AIDS

Mary Tasker, M.S.W.

Managing Editor:
  Elizabeth Seale Jeppson, Ph.D.

Illustrator:
  Katherine VanHorne
  Piedmont, California

ASSOCIATION FOR THE CARE OF CHILDREN'S HEALTH
BETHESDA, MARYLAND

Published by Association for the Care of Children's Health
7910 Woodmont Avenue, Suite 300
Bethesda, MD 20814

Additional copies are available for purchase from the publisher.

ISBN 0-937821-82-9

Dedication

This is essentially a book about some very special families. However, there is one family above all whose unstinting love and support have made this book possible. That family is my own.

Eugene Lieber — my husband and friend. His unwavering belief in the work I do, regardless of the time or energy it commands, is inspirational and nurturing. He is a true feminist.

Simon Tasker — the self-discipline in his own life encourages me to go on when energy is low. His extreme good nature lifts my sad moods while his gentle teasing of my intensity keeps me grounded.

Michael Tasker — his commitment to a politics of inclusion, rather than the exclusionary version currently in vogue, has taught me much. His capacity for forgiveness and acceptance of limitations in others is a model for me.

Preface

In many ways, I began writing this book six years ago when I first started working with HIV-infected children and their families. At that time, very few of the children served by our multi-disciplinary team seemed aware of their diagnosis — the secret was so tightly guarded by their parents. It seemed to us that the reasons parents kept the secret of AIDS were perfectly understandable, given the hysteria and discriminatory attitudes in society, and the growing number of incidents of hostility and aggression towards people with AIDS, including children and families. The issue of disclosing the diagnosis to children did not appear urgent; it seemed that once children became infected with the virus, their lifespans were very short.

However, new treatments began to offer new hope, for adults and also children. Children were surviving longer, and entering the school system. Additionally, an increasing number of children were being identified for the first time at 5, 6, and 7 years of age. Many of these children had been infected during the perinatal period, but had passed their earliest years relatively symptom free. The issue of talking to children about their diagnosis became increasingly relevant. Also, in families where no children were actually infected, there were the many hundreds of children to consider who were affected by the diagnosis of an adult family member.

It was in this context that I first began to explore with parents the issues around disclosing the diagnosis to children. I also began to talk about the issues of secrecy and disclosure whenever I appeared before my professional colleagues. During these seminars, I stated what I do not state anywhere in this book: that my own bias as a professional was that children should be told their diagnosis. However, I always said and believed in the caveat "but not without the consent and participation of their parents." Although in my daily practice and interactions with parents, I frequently raised the topic of telling children the diagnosis, there was never any doubt in my mind that all authority in this decision-making process rested with the parent.

Just over two years ago at the 5th Annual National Pediatric AIDS Conference in Los Angeles, I was asked to present on this topic. The audience consisted of both parents and professionals, and it was the first time I had given the talk to such a group. Many of the parents I knew from my own practice were in the audience, and they were generally supportive. However, I clearly remember parents from other areas of the country challenging, with tremendous passion and eloquence, my assertions that children should be told their diagnosis.

As I began working on this book, two incidents happened that, I believe, significantly altered the way this book is written. The first was an encounter I had with a professional colleague as we left the funeral of a child we had both known. She told me that she had heard I was working on a book about disclosure, and asked me if it was still my position that parents "have got to tell their children the diagnosis." I was both shocked and dismayed at this characterization of my position on the issues, and I responded that I had never made that assertion. I told her that the book was about issues of secrecy and disclosure, and although my professional bias was that it was better for children to be told their diagnosis, I certainly did not believe that parents must tell their children.

The second encounter was with a mother I met during an ACCH Family Network Meeting. She introduced herself and said she was one of the parents who had challenged me at the Pediatric AIDS Conference in Los Angeles. She spoke to me about the dangers of disclosing the diagnosis, particularly her fears about acts of aggression toward families when the child's diagnosis became known. She also talked about the extraordinary stresses of keeping the secret. As our conversation continued, she told me that in my workshop presentation in Los Angeles, I had come across as the "caped crusader of telling" (the diagnosis). She commented that she was pleasantly surprised to find that in person I was far more open on the issue, and appeared to show much more empathy to a parent's decision not to tell.

Both of these experiences had a profound impact on me and on the writing of this book, which was already underway. As I reviewed the first draft outlines of the book with my ACCH colleagues and mentors, I could see that the style and structure of the writing seemed to convey a one-sided view toward disclosure. This was never my intention or my philosophy. And so gradually the style and form of the book began to change into its present form, which more closely follows the beliefs and practices I have always had as a social worker — that parents know their children best, and it is their wisdom and knowledge that should guide professional practice.

As I attempt to illustrate throughout this book, the issues of secrecy and disclosure of an AIDS diagnosis to children are profound and complex. Further, they are not static issues. When a parent makes a decision to keep the secret, that decision is made at a particular moment in time under a very specific set of circumstances. Times change, circumstances change, and so, too, do parents' feelings about disclosure. The process of deciding to tell or not to tell is ongoing. Families bring wisdom and strength to the process, and each family identifies its own set of criteria about whom, when, and what they will and will not tell.

Over the years, I have found that despite all the obstacles to telling, many parents do eventually decide to disclose the diagnosis. And much of the research I have done indicates that the majority feel a great sense of relief when they do. But again, it is the family who must decide, for they are the ones who will live with the consequences of the decision.

The collective wisdom of many, many parents caring for children infected or affected by HIV has shaped and reshaped this book. Their experiences and stories have much to teach us. For all they have taught me, I thank them.

Mary Tasker, M.S.W.
Montclair, New Jersey
February 1992

Introduction

As of December 31, 1991, a total of 3,471 cases of AIDS in children under the age of 13 had been reported to the Centers for Disease Control (CDC). It is widely accepted in the health care field that this figure is only the tip of the iceberg, reflecting but a tiny portion of the HIV epidemic. Some experts believe there may be as many as ten children who are HIV infected for every child actually diagnosed with AIDS. In addition to the growing number of children infected with HIV, there are many thousands of children profoundly affected by the impact of HIV/AIDS on a close family member — a mother, father, sibling, or other relative in the kinship network.

HIV/AIDS is not only a medical problem. It is also a social problem, and the diagnosis carries a stigma that has profound psychological, social, and emotional ramifications. For this reason when a person is HIV infected, the diagnosis is often a closely guarded secret — even within the family. And children, even when they are infected, are often the last to whom the diagnosis is disclosed.

The issue of educating children about AIDS is being widely discussed in this country. Policy makers, educators, and parents are struggling with difficult questions. Should children be educated about AIDS? How should they be told? Who should tell them? At what age should AIDS be discussed? In what setting — home or school? What should we tell children about AIDS? Do we call it a fatal illness or a chronic disease? How will they react to the knowledge that not only adults but also children can be HIV infected? How can we help them with the fears they may have?

These questions are even more complex when children or their parents or brothers and sisters are HIV infected. To date, these issues have received very little attention in the professional literature and yet they are being confronted or avoided in the many homes, clinics, and hospitals where families affected by HIV/AIDS seek care and support. Thousands of parents and the professionals with whom they work are struggling with these disturbing questions on a daily basis.

This publication has been developed to assist families and professionals as they explore the complex and diverse issues that surround the disclosure of the HIV diagnosis to children. It is a work that draws from a variety of sources, and is grounded in the experience of the many families and professionals in the Newark, New Jersey, area with whom the author has been privileged to work for the past six years. Other material has been gathered from the families the author has come to know through the ACCH Family Network.

If the readers of this publication draw inspiration, insight, and renewed conviction to work on behalf of children and families faced with a diagnosis of HIV/AIDS, all thanks are due to the courageous families and dedicated professionals who have so generously shared their struggles and experiences. Their stories teach us; they inspire us by their example.

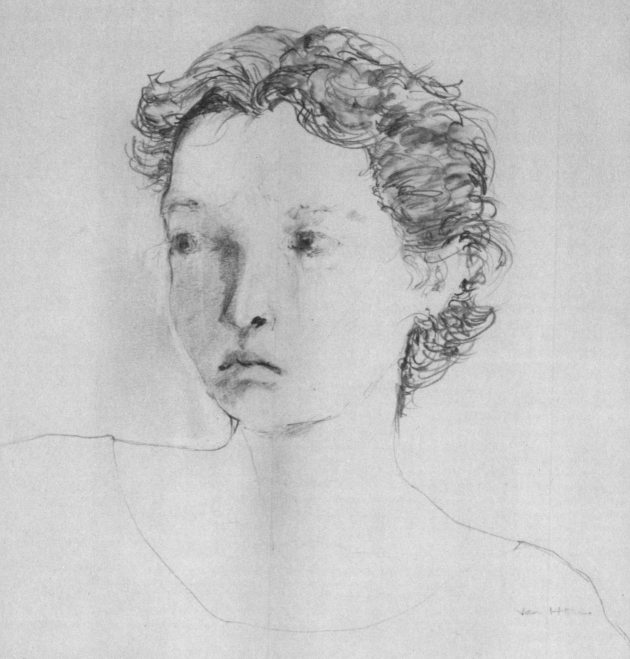

It seems to me you could die of a broken heart
before AIDS even gets a chance to kill you.

CHAPTER I

HIV/AIDS:
A Closely Guarded Secret

The first thought most adults have upon learning that a family member is HIV infected is that the diagnosis must be kept a very closely guarded secret. They make initial vows never to disclose the diagnosis to *anyone*. After some period of time — this may be hours, weeks, months, or longer — they may choose to share the knowledge with one or more trusted people. For the majority of families, however, keeping the secret of AIDS becomes a way of life. Although it is stressful, burdensome, and lonely, there are many legitimate reasons why they choose to be the guardians of the secret of AIDS.

The Unpredictable Nature of the Response

The reason family members most often cite for their reluctance to disclose the diagnosis is their fear of the reaction of others.

JENNIFER IS THE MOTHER of 20-month-old Peter and 6-year-old Nicole. Since birth, Peter has suffered from a variety of upper respiratory infections and skin rashes. During one hospitalization, Jennifer agreed to have Peter tested for HIV infection. She was told that he was HIV positive. At a later date, Jennifer describes herself as "being in a fog" for two weeks following the diagnosis. As she came out of this fog, she recalls being asked by the doctors if she had told her family Peter's diagnosis. She replied that she had not and, furthermore, that she would not.

Jennifer: "How could I tell them when I didn't know what their reaction would be? I thought they would shut the door on me or maybe disown me. There was no way I could even think about telling them if I didn't know how they would take it."

Jennifer's fears are not unfounded. In the early years of the epidemic there were many cases of discrimination against HIV-infected individuals and their family members. In one case, the uninfected brother of an HIV-infected child was barred from returning to school once his sister's diagnosis became known. It took legal action to obtain the boy's re-entry into the school system. His foster mother describes her shock at this unexpected reaction by educators.

Foster mother: "I had told the principal about my daughter's diagnosis in confidence. I chose to tell him first because, being so educated, I felt he would not react in the crazy way that many other people have when they heard 'AIDS.' Also, my son had already been in the school for two years and it had been a very good experience. I had always admired the way the principal had run things. I was so shocked the day my son came home from school with a note that said he could not return because he might pose a threat. My son didn't even have the virus. I couldn't believe that these educated people were acting in such an hysterical way."

The Potential Loss of Valued People

The unpredictable nature of the response causes many adults to keep the secret of HIV/AIDS from others who may possibly discriminate or retaliate against them. They also withhold the diagnosis because they do not wish to risk losing the support of a valued family member or close friend.

EVA IS THE MATERNAL GRANDMOTHER and legal guardian of Jameel, who is 14, and 4-year-old Kiyah. Eva took over the care of her grandchildren several months prior to the death of her daughter, Liah. When it was time for Eva to return to her job, she placed Kiyah in the care of Emma, an old family friend. Emma had taken care of Liah when she was a child; she was almost an institution in the family. Eva had struggled hard with her decision not to tell Emma that Kiyah was HIV infected.

Eva: "I trusted Emma a great deal but I felt I could not tell her the diagnosis. There was so much stigma attached to AIDS and no way you could predict how anyone would react. Certainly I knew the doctors felt I should tell her, and it did play on my conscience *not* to tell. But I just did not feel comfortable telling her. She had been around our family for many years. She was very important to me. She had taken care of my daughter, Liah, when she was a child. I just could not bear the thought of losing her."

While many parents might feel able to withstand the effects of social rejection themselves, they would find it intolerable for their children.

DIANE IS THE MOTHER of 11-year-old Missy and 2-year-old Shanell who is HIV infected. Diane talks about her decision not to tell her own father that she and Shanell are infected.

Diane: "I know it would be very hard for me if I told my father I have AIDS and he rejected me. Last night I read in the paper where the parents of this gay man would not even come to his hospital bed when he was dying. Maybe I could even stand it for myself, but if he rejected Shanell I know it would be more than I could bear. It seems to me, when I think about it, that you could die from a broken heart, before AIDS even gets a chance to kill you, if your own parents were afraid to hold your child in their arms."

Fears the Child Will Disclose the Diagnosis to Others

Despite initial vows not to disclose the diagnosis to anyone, most adults gradually begin to take others into their confidence. Children, however, are usually the last to be told that a family member has AIDS. This family secret is also kept from children who are themselves HIV infected or have AIDS. Perhaps the most frequently cited reason for not telling children the diagnosis is the fear the child will disclose the diagnosis to others.

> CARMEN IS THE FOSTER MOTHER of Lisette, age 9, and 12-year-old David. Carmen is in the process of adopting the siblings. Lisette is HIV infected and mildly symptomatic. Lisette's health care team has suggested to Carmen that she reveal the diagnosis to Lisette. Carmen feels this is impossible.

> *Carmen:* "How could I possibly tell Lisette that she has the AIDS virus? It would be all over town the next day. The doctor thinks Lisette is old enough to learn to keep this secret, but she doesn't know Lisette. In spite of the way I have tried to raise her, Lisette is very impulsive. I have to even say she is a blabbermouth. It seems like she cannot keep anything to herself. I know I could tell David that his sister has the virus and he would keep it private. If I told Lisette she would probably tell everyone on our block and at school, then who knows what would happen. Maybe they would burn my house down. At the least she would probably have no more friends at school. No, I cannot tell Lisette because she will tell the world."

A physician working with families affected by HIV expresses understanding of the vulnerable position that families put themselves in when they reveal the diagnosis to a child.

> *Physician:* "One night my husband came home very late from a business trip and, so as not to disturb me, he slept in our guest room. The next day my son told my mother-in-law that 'Daddy sleeps in the guest room.' My mother-in-law called my husband and asked him if we were having marital problems, and it took a lot of convincing to explain to her that everything was all right. This was such a little incident, and it had such a big impact. Can you imagine what we are asking families to risk exposing themselves to when we suggest they should tell children that someone in their family has AIDS?"

One Thing Leads to Another

Keeping the secret of AIDS from children may also mean keeping other secrets from them. When a parent becomes infected through drug use and the sharing of needles, disclosing the diagnosis means risking the child will discover how the parent became infected. Many parents feel they would not be able to answer their children's questions about their drug use. Few parents believe their child would be able to understand addiction as a disease and would instead see the parent as a bad person.

In contemplating the impact of disclosing her diagnosis to her oldest daughter, Nicole, Jennifer speaks about her fears of facing Nicole's questions.

Jennifer: "Nicole is a very bright child and she has a lot of curiosity. If I tell her that her mommy and daddy both have the AIDS virus, she is not just going to leave it at that. Pretty soon she will be asking how we got it. There is no way that I can tell her what we have without it leading to more questions that I do not want to answer. Even though she is very intelligent, she is still a child with a child's thinking. I can't even think of telling my own family and they are adults. Whenever the adults in my family talk about AIDS, they talk about it as if it were a dirty word — as if it were a curse. In their eyes, only certain types of people get AIDS — drug addicts and prostitutes. Always they think of it as something bad people get. Someone who is a drug addict is simply a bad person. It is not possible for them to think of a drug addict as a human being with a problem. If they are mature adults and they think that way, how can I possibly explain it to Nicole so that she will understand?"

Other parents share Jennifer's concern that disclosing the diagnosis will lead to further questions that are both painful and difficult to answer.

LISA IS THE MOTHER of 9-year-old Monique and 8-month-old Joey. Lisa is HIV infected but symptom free. She feels fortunate that neither of her children is infected. Lisa often imagines the day she might have to tell Monique her diagnosis and she worries about the kinds of questions

Monique will have. During a visit to her doctor, Lisa was asked about her reservations in telling Monique. Lisa shares her fears that Monique will ask too many questions.

Lisa: "If I tell Monique that I have the AIDS virus I know she will have many questions. She is an intelligent girl and she knows a lot about AIDS. I have helped her to be well informed. She knows how people can become HIV infected. I am sure she would be very curious and want to know how I became infected. One question would lead to another and I don't know how I would answer her."

The Stigma of AIDS

The word stigma originates from the Greek word for a mark or tatoo. In English it describes an attribute that is deeply discrediting. Parents fear that the stigma of AIDS will have a widespread negative impact on their children and their families. In fact, the power of the stigma attached to the very word AIDS is so great that many family members have difficulty saying it aloud. Euphemisms like "the disease," "that virus," or "his illness" are often substituted, as if the mere mention of the word could bring about harm. The words of a psychologist working with the mother of a child with HIV infection illustrate this point.

Psychologist: "Every time Laurie's mother wants to discuss the effects of HIV infection on her daughter's growth and development, she simply cannot say the word AIDS or HIV. She refers to it as 'Laurie's illness,' or infection. I can feel the power that the word AIDS has over her, and when I am in her presence I keep thinking of Hawthorne's novel, *The Scarlet Letter*. It is as if Laurie and her mother are both branded with an invisible letter 'A' on their foreheads and they fear that saying the word, even in private, will make it possible for other people to become aware of it."

Even when parents have not used drugs, they fear their children associate the disease with being bad or doing bad things. Parents often cite the influence of negative stereotypes in society at large, and particularly the influence of television, in shaping their children's assumptions about the types of people who get AIDS.

Responsibility to Protect the Child

Another reason that parents cite for not revealing the diagnosis is the responsibility they feel to protect the child from harm, and from the stress of hearing traumatic news. Parents often say they feel the child is better off not knowing.

> LISA HAS KNOWN about her diagnosis for four years, but has chosen not to tell Monique. Lisa describes Monique as a happy, confident, outgoing child who does well in school and has many friends. Lisa's social worker at the hospital asks her why she has chosen not to tell Monique.
>
> *Lisa:* "The main reason I don't tell is because I don't see a need to tell. My own health is good. If a miracle happened and they found a cure, I would never have to tell. The most important reason I don't tell is that it would put a lot of pressure on her. She's doing very well in life. She's happy and really enjoys school. If she knew, it would be a burden. She would associate AIDS with death and then she wouldn't be hopeful. She is much better off not knowing."
>
> FOR JOAN, THE MOTHER of 12-year-old Michael and 7-year-old Melissa, the decision not to tell is based on her desire to protect her children from a traumatic reality. Melissa is HIV infected but asymptomatic. Joan states that she feels Melissa is too young to know her diagnosis, and although she has considered telling Michael about his sister, she has dismissed the idea.
>
> *Joan:* "It really didn't take me very long to decide that I would not tell Michael about Melissa. Why should I disrupt his childhood? I don't want him to have to bear the burden of keeping the secret like I do. Keeping this secret is not an easy task. You have to be constantly on guard so

that you don't slip up. I have found it so difficult to lie. I even found myself staying away from many of my friends in case I accidentally let something slip. I certainly avoided making new friends. The stress of it caused me to overeat and I put on 30 pounds. I think, in a way, putting on that extra weight was like creating an extra boundary or buffer around myself to keep people away. If it is so difficult for me and so stressful, why would I subject Michael to that? I feel it is my duty as a parent to protect my children as long as I can and allow them to live a normal, happy life."

Parents may also decide to delay disclosing the diagnosis until the timing and circumstances are right.

DANA IS THE MOTHER of 12-year-old Alicia and 11-year-old Omar. Dana feels strongly that there should be few secrets between herself and her children, but for two years after learning her own diagnosis, she did not share it with them.

Dana: "The fact that I am HIV infected is definitely something I feel they should know, but the timing needs to be right. At the time I first learned I was infected, Alicia and Omar were having a lot of difficulties. They had just returned from spending the whole summer with their grandmother, aunts, and cousins in California, and had to face the fact that, while they were away, their father had deserted us. It was a very painful time for us all. Also, I had to break the news to them that I had had a miscarriage, perhaps because of all the stress. This made them both very sad since they had been excited about having a new baby brother or sister. It was a lot of losses for them at one time. In addition, they had lived a kind of wild and undisciplined life for the summer, surrounded by many relatives, and they now had to adjust to the discipline of returning to school and our quiet home. It took them a long time to adjust and get back to normal.

"When they first returned they were often depressed and tearful, and we all felt the tension. How could I have possibly told them at this time? What a tremendous burden this would have placed on their shoulders. Sure, there were many times when I wanted to tell them because we had always been so close and I was not used to keeping important information from them. I'm sure that in telling them I would have felt some relief. But what kind of parent would that have made me? No, I had to give them time to make their adjustment, to regain confidence and trust. They would need to have a lot more strength before I could ask them to face more difficulties."

Fears About Discussing Death With Children

Although treatment for the manifestations of HIV/AIDS has improved over the past five years, it is a painful fact that there is no known cure. Therefore, many families make an automatic link between AIDS and death when a loved one is infected. One parent describes this connection in a very dramatic way.

> *Parent:* "I remember not only the day my daughter was diagnosed, but also the exact moment in time. I was looking at the clock just before the doctor stepped into the room. It was 2:35 p.m. By the time it was 2:45 p.m., I knew my daughter had AIDS. Therefore, I knew I had it also, and I guessed my husband had it since he was the one who used drugs. So at 2:45 p.m., I knew that my whole family was going to die."

Faced with this knowledge, many parents feel that it would be impossible to tell a child that she or another family member has AIDS without also confronting the child's fears about death.

> ALLISA IS THE ADOPTIVE MOTHER of 9-year-old Keesha who is HIV infected. Allisa is struggling with the issue of telling Keesha her diagnosis, but has been unable to come to terms with all of the implications of telling.

> *Allisa:* "It's one thing to talk about HIV and another thing to talk about AIDS. If you could just say HIV and leave it at that, maybe it wouldn't seem so difficult. When there are programs on TV, nobody talks about HIV and death. It is always AIDS and death. They say 'a man with AIDS died; a woman with AIDS died; a child with AIDS died.' They don't say anyone died of HIV. If, somehow, Keesha would

not automatically associate AIDS with death, it might be possible for me to say AIDS to her. But I'm afraid she would hear AIDS and think 'you get wrinkled up and you die.' You see, it's not just that she associates AIDS with death, but also, because of the type of stories they have on TV, she would remember the stories they have shown of people wasting away and dying. I realize that they probably always show the most frightening, drastic cases this way to try and make a point, maybe to get people to use condoms, but it doesn't give any room for hope. AIDS is associated with a really horrible way to die, and I cannot imagine how I would be able to deal with this image of death with Keesha."

There are many compelling reasons why families keep the diagnosis a closely guarded secret; yet the burden of keeping this secret is enormous. Most of the families whose stories are told in this chapter talk about the complexity involved in maintaining secrecy, including the necessity to lie. One parent sums it up in the following way.

Parent: "Keeping this secret means constantly telling lies. This goes against your own moral code, and your conscience is often troubled by it. It is also *very* stressful; you have to remember who you told and what it was that you said to them. You have to become intentionally schizophrenic. You find yourself often terrified that you will slip and say something to someone who might give something away. So in a way you are always on guard, thinking about everything you say before you open your mouth. Pretty soon you find yourself avoiding people because it is too much work to be constantly having to watch yourself and what you say. It's not natural. But you force it to become your second nature, because the price you might have to pay for telling could be too great. A lot of professionals feel we should tell our children, and we often feel that way, too. In the best of all possible worlds, we would not have to live this way. But this is not the best of all possible worlds, and we are the ones who have to face that."

Chapter Summary

Many parents' first reaction upon learning that a family member has AIDS is to not tell anyone, particularly because the nature of the response to disclosure is so unpredictable. Parents fear the loss of, or rejection by, valued friends or family members, and especially want to protect their child from this experience.

The reluctance to tell a child the diagnosis may be based on fears that the child will disclose the diagnosis to others, resulting in negative repercussions for the family. Parents are also concerned that once children know the diagnosis, they will be curious about how the family member became infected; this, in turn, could lead to further questions about parental drug use or sexual behavior. Many parents feel that children believe that only bad people get AIDS and that answering children's questions on these issues would be difficult and embarrassing.

Parents may withhold the diagnosis in order to protect their children from painful realities and to preserve and maintain happy childhood experiences for as long as possible. Even when parents have a strong wish to tell, they may delay disclosure if children are struggling with other difficult family or developmental issues, thus giving the child needed time to adjust.

Due to the tendency to link AIDS and death, parents are concerned that disclosing the diagnosis will also mean talking to their child about death. Many parents feel unprepared to face this awesome responsibility, particularly since the graphic depiction of AIDS-related deaths on television may leave frightening images in children's minds.

Despite the legitimate reasons to keep the diagnosis a closely guarded secret, many parents yearn to leave the world of concealment and lies, a world often in conflict with their own moral values. They look forward to a time when they will be free of the tremendously painful existence of living in the shadows with AIDS.

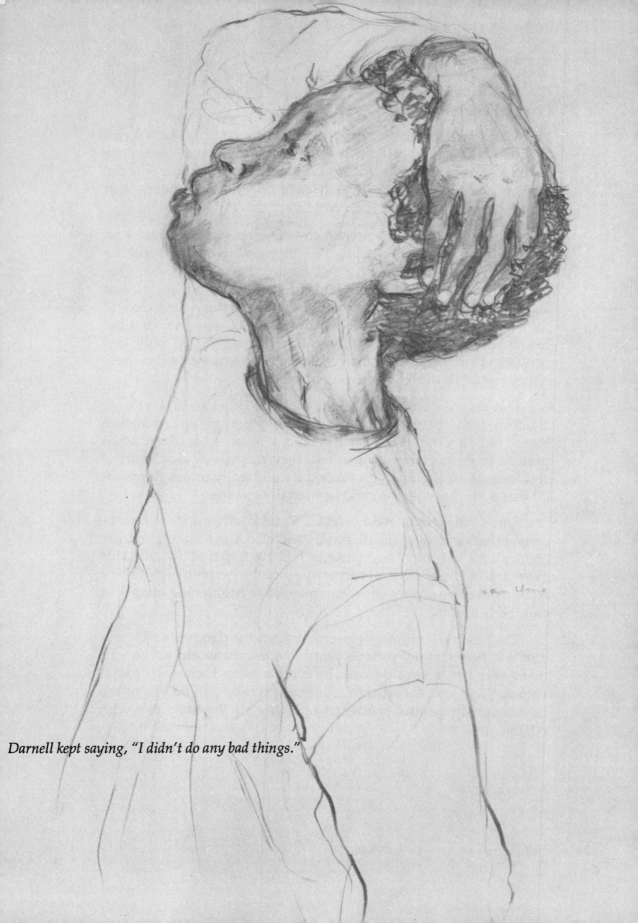

Darnell kept saying, "I didn't do any bad things."

CHAPTER II

The Burden of Secrecy

Although there are many powerful reasons for not revealing the diagnosis of HIV/AIDS to children, there are also stresses and risks involved in keeping the secret.

Dana: "Unless you have lived with this secret as long as I have, you cannot possibly imagine just how difficult it is to keep the secret to yourself. At the time I was diagnosed, it seemed like everyone I met was constantly talking about AIDS. One time, I was with some of my friends and they were all agreeing that you could tell that a person had AIDS just by looking at them. I guess they thought people with AIDS were abnormal looking. I wanted to blurt out that I was positive, to prove them wrong. It drove me crazy that I couldn't tell them, but I forced myself to keep quiet because who knows where it would lead to if I told them?

"Keeping quiet about the fact that you are infected is the hardest thing you have to do. It is like cutting off part of you inside. It hurts so much not being able to be me. You have to learn to be two people. You may be having a general conversation with another person and then the topic switches to AIDS. You have to respond as if the subject of AIDS is as neutral to you as it is to them, when the truth is you are wanting with all your heart to tell them that you have it. But you can't tell them, so you have to tighten the lid on your secret and it builds up inside like a pressure cooker. When this happens to me it seems as if my heart is pounding, I feel hot and sweaty, and there is a knot in the pit of my stomach. You would think all of this would be noticeable to the other person, but they just go on talking as if the world is normal. That's when you know that you have learned to turn into a completely different person, one who looks normal on the outside, but is crumbling to pieces inside."

In addition to the personal stress and loneliness that result from keeping the diagnosis secret, research suggests that secrets within families, particularly those between parents and children, can have a very negative impact.

> There should be no secrets. Secrets isolate the child and increase the likelihood that the child will hear the information and it may not be accurate. Secrets create distrust between the child and caregivers. . . . Energy is expended in protecting information and this distorts meaningful communication within the family while limiting any chance for maintaining a reasonably normal life. (Pearson, 1981)

There is also evidence that in spite of parental efforts, children often come to know their diagnosis without ever being expressly told. This phenomenon, which is reported in the literature on children with other life-threatening conditions, suggests that it is probably impossible to protect children from the diagnosis indefinitely (Spinetta & Deasy-Spinetta, 1980). The parents of a boy with HIV infection speak of what they consider to be the "myth" that children do not know.

> ANDREW IS THE BIRTH FATHER of Larry, 15, and Joel, 7. Simone is his second wife, to whom he has been married for two years. Joel is HIV positive and symptomatic, although he maintains good health and is in school. Both he and his older brother Larry are aware of his diagnosis. The parents decided early on that it would be almost impossible to shield the diagnosis from Joel. The parents often encourage other parents to tell children their diagnosis.

> *Simone:* "Every month we bring our children to this clinic, and they sit here for three hours or more connected to their IVs with a room full of other kids and parents."

Andrew: "Yes. Everyone knows this is a clinic for kids with AIDS. There is no real privacy here. Even if the adults don't say the word AIDS, all day long they are talking about PCP and AZT."

Simone: "Do they think these kids are deaf or stupid? They watch TV. They hear these words and they know these words are connected with AIDS. We are all kidding ourselves if we think they do not know what is going on. The more we try and keep this thing a secret, the more they will try and find out what is going on, and the more they will resent us for not telling them what is going on with their own bodies."

If a child has not been told the diagnosis but comes to know it anyway, she may harbor bitter resentments that distort future interactions with the adults guarding the secret. Two adolescent boys face this situation as their parents remain locked in their commitment to keep the secret of AIDS.

BOTH PARENTS ARE ILL. The father is in the intensive care unit of a nearby hospital, and the mother is so debilitated by infections associated with AIDS that she can no longer visit her husband's bedside. However, she refuses to let her sons visit without her supervision; she is afraid that hospital personnel, unwittingly or otherwise, will reveal the diagnosis to them. The boys are not allowed to visit their father, nor are they given any means to work out their feelings. The boys begin aggressive acting-out, both at home and at school. Their emotional development becomes stunted as they are locked out of the family's inner circle. A social worker assigned to the family through a home care agency has been unable to convince the mother that the behavior of both boys might be tied to their being denied access to the family secret, and their resulting anger. In consultation with her supervisor, the social worker describes the situation.

Social worker: "I just know they have guessed what the big secret is and they are furious with their mother for not respecting their right to know. They feel it means she doesn't trust them. They make insulting references to their mother 'treating them like babies' in my presence. They ask me leading questions in her presence, but she has forbidden me to tell them anything. She tells me they have begun to talk a lot about people with AIDS and she is shocked by the kinds of things they say. She was broken-hearted recently when one of the boys told her he thought that all people who have AIDS should be branded like cattle so you could identify them. She feels they *mean* this and that they hold the same negative ideas about people with AIDS as some of the more sensational media types. This reinforces her decision not to tell them. I feel they are provoking her, they are just screaming out to her in their anger and their pain 'please tell us what we already know.'"

Parents do sometimes discover that their children have known about the diagnosis even though they were not expressly told. When this happens, parents may regret that they did not disclose the diagnosis. One parent relates the story of the day she discovered that her child already knew the family secret.

MARILYN NOTICED that her daughter Aimee was unusually quiet on the ride home from school. Ordinarily, Aimee was eager to tell her mother all the new things she was learning in school each day. Perhaps, Marilyn thought, Aimee was reflecting on some new and fascinating knowledge. As if to confirm her mother's speculations, Aimee pierced through the silence asking, "Mommy, do you know that children can get AIDS and not just grown-ups?" Marilyn replied that she did know this. Aimee continued, "Do *you* know any kids who have AIDS?" Swallowing hard, Marilyn replied that she did not personally know any children who had AIDS. A long silence ensued, then once again Aimee broke it abruptly. "Mommy, do you ever tell lies?" Believing that her daughter had changed topics, Marilyn responded that she always tried to tell the truth. At this point Aimee burst into tears and sobbed, "No you don't. You told me my sister died of cancer, but she had AIDS and you have it, too!"

Just as some children like Aimee gradually become aware of the AIDS diagnosis, others learn the diagnosis in an abrupt and often shocking way. Such incidents may leave a parent or guardian with deep feelings of regret.

LOUISE IS THE GRANDMOTHER AND LEGAL GUARDIAN of 13-year-old Stanley and 7-year-old Darnell. Darnell has AIDS, but his health has been relatively stable. Louise felt that Stanley was old enough to be told about his brother's diagnosis, but that Darnell was still too young to understand. Whenever Darnell asks about why he needs to go to the clinic, he is given an explanation related to his current symptoms, rather than told he has AIDS. Louise is uncertain that Darnell is either ready or mature enough to handle knowing his real diagnosis. However, she later regrets not disclosing the diagnosis herself, as Darnell comes to know it in an unexpected turn of events.

Louise: "Stanley had been to his doctor for a check-up and was outside talking to his friends. As these teenagers sometimes do, the other boys began teasing Stanley about his great interest in girls. Apparently, one of the boys began to say that Stanley had gone for a check-up because he had V.D. Kids are pretty mean sometimes, and soon everyone was chanting 'Stanley has V.D. Stanley has V.D.' Even though Darnell didn't know what *that* was, I guess he thought he would join in with the big boys, so he began to chant it, too. Pretty soon Stanley got mad and yelled something at Darnell. I didn't know what it was, until Darnell came running in to me crying, and told me that Stanley had told him, 'So what, you go to the clinic because you've got AIDS.'

"Darnell was hysterical at first, and even when I got him calmed down, he was still pretty upset. I knew I couldn't lie to him anymore, so I tried to explain it to him. He kept saying 'I didn't do any bad things.' When we talked some more it was clear he had heard some stories about AIDS on the television, and in his mind he associated having AIDS with doing bad things. I decided that I would like some help in explaining it all to him properly, so I called up his doctor and made an appointment. I didn't want Darnell to think that he had done anything bad. I really regretted he had found out in this way, and I wished that I had told him myself much earlier. I feared it would take a lot of work to undo the harm that had been done by learning it in this way. Also, now other children on the block knew, so I knew it wouldn't be too long before they told their parents."

As Louise discovered, there are risks for a parent in not disclosing the diagnosis to a child. Perhaps chief among them is that the child will learn the diagnosis under undesirable circumstances. But it is not only to avoid such accidental disclosures that parents decide to discuss the diagnosis with their children. There are also benefits to disclosure.

Benefits of Disclosure

First, open and honest discussions between adults and children promote growth — intellectual as well as emotional. An environment that supports communication among family members enhances a child's ability to cope.

> The opportunity to help a child face reality and handle his deep emotions wisely is a privilege to be treasured. It invites the care and competence of one who is deeply concerned with both the immediate and long-term results. When this help is given, the child moves into his future better equipped for life. Though he may not know it or be able to express it adequately, he owes a debt of gratitude to the adults who have wisely furnished him with sound resources for his inner development. (Jackson, 1965, p. 78)

Parents of children affected by HIV and AIDS have stated that their children behaved more maturely and responsibly after learning the diagnosis.

Andrew: "It was Simone who convinced me that Larry was old enough to know about his brother's diagnosis. I wasn't sure she was right, but she talked me into it. Larry was always asking me about why Joel had to go to the clinic and get all the needles and the medicine, and I kept telling him it was because Joel had weak lungs when he was little, but I knew my explanation didn't satisfy him. So, I decided to trust Simone's judgment and tell him. Naturally he was shocked and very upset. But I have to say that Simone proved to be right on this. Once Larry knew, he tried to be a lot more understanding towards Joel, especially on clinic days when Joel was often cranky. Also, Larry began to tell us that Joel would be able to fight this thing because he had the best family in the world. He would cheer Simone and me up when we were feeling down. I think it made him feel like he was a real man in the house because he knew we had shown our respect for his maturity, and he also knew how much we relied on his support in caring for Joel."

Second, in spite of parental concerns that knowledge of the diagnosis will increase the child's fears, the literature indicates otherwise (Kellerman, Rigler, Siegel, & Katz, 1977). Telling a child the diagnosis and prognosis permits the child to talk openly about his feelings.

> Giving the child such opportunities does not heighten death anxiety; on the contrary, understanding acceptance and conveyance of permission to discuss any aspects of his illness may decrease feelings of isolation, alienation, and the sense that his illness is too terrible to discuss completely. (Waechter, 1971, p. 1171)

The opportunity to discuss the diagnosis and its implications can also help children and other family members develop strategies for living with the AIDS virus. With advances in early diagnosis and treatment, particularly the availability of antiviral therapies, the life expectancy of people infected with HIV is increasing and AIDS is beginning to be considered a chronic illness.

Dana: "My first reaction to learning that I was HIV infected was to think about death. All that rang in my mind was AIDS and death. It took a long time for me to understand that being HIV infected was not the same as having AIDS, and that having AIDS did not mean I would die the next day. In other words, it took a lot of time and the hard work of the doctors and nurses at the clinic to make me believe there was hope, that I could *live* with the AIDS virus.

"Once I got this into my head and settled down to living, I
began to think about HIV as a chronic condition, which is
what my doctor called it. For me, this meant becoming
serious about eating right, getting exercise without
overdoing it, and getting plenty of rest. Most importantly,
it meant staying in a good place in my head and believing I
can beat this thing. A good attitude and fighting spirit are
as important to my health as AZT."

Parents of children who are HIV infected are also beginning
to anticipate helping their children survive on a long-term basis.
As they begin to view HIV as a chronic condition, their optimism
leads them to reconsider the issue of disclosing the diagnosis.

Allisa: "For years I have felt that I could not tell Keesha the
diagnosis. Certainly I have a lot of anxiety when I think
about answering her questions about death. But in the past
I used to think that I would only have Keesha for a few
short years. Now I have gone five years over what I
thought would be the limit for her life. She is still doing so
well. Maybe I will go ten years over the limit with her. I
have started to think about her becoming a teenager, and to
imagine her going out on dates. What if she became
sexually active? No matter what you may feel about it,
teenagers sometimes make their own decisions. I cannot be
behind her all the time, checking up on her, cautioning her.
When she is older she will have to have more freedom, and
naturally that means she will have to know her diagnosis.
If she did not know it, how would she make responsible
and informed decisions?"

Chapter Summary

Although many adults vow never to reveal the diagnosis, the
burden and risks of living with the secret can be overwhelming.
The energy required to maintain secrecy creates distrust and tension in a family. Further, in spite of efforts to protect children from
knowing the diagnosis, they often come to know it whether or not
deliberately told by a trusted adult. When a child accidentally discovers that she or a family member is HIV infected, she may be

deeply hurt and frightened and parents often regret not having been in control of the disclosure issue.

There are also benefits to disclosure. The child's emotional and intellectual development and his ability to cope with the stresses of illness may be enhanced by the opportunity to talk openly with adult family members. The child's fears and sense of isolation are also reduced in an atmosphere of open communication. This climate of openness can help both the child and family develop more effective strategies for living with a chronic illness.

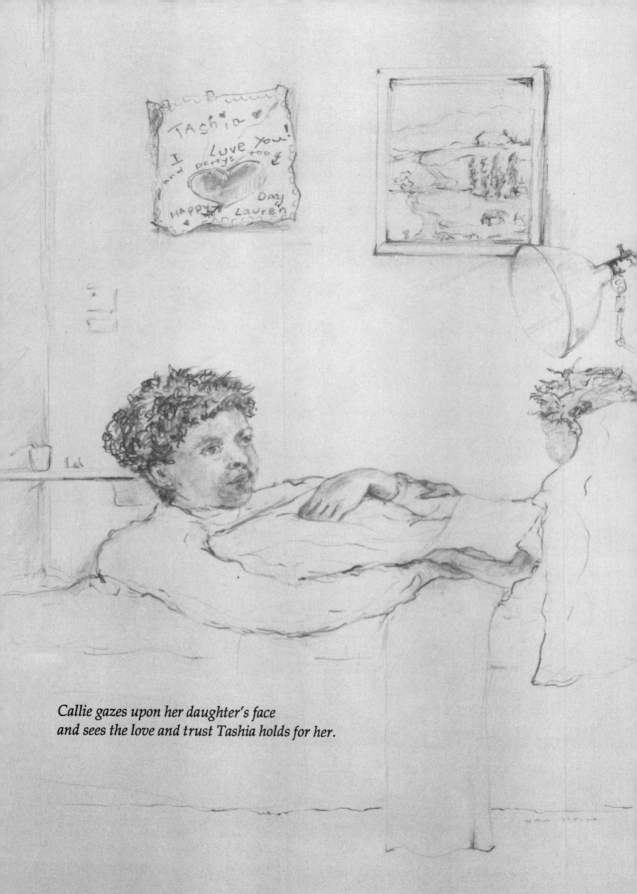

Callie gazes upon her daughter's face
and sees the love and trust Tashia holds for her.

CHAPTER III

Stigma and Discrimination: Barriers to Disclosure

Individuals who test positive for HIV are potentially subject to at least two types of discrimination. First, they carry a virus that is regarded with dread because of its virulence; and second, this virus and the diseases associated with it are connected, at least in the popular imagination, with socially marginal groups such as gay men, intravenous drug users, and blacks and Hispanics. From an external point of view, if not from their own perspective, HIV-infected individuals are metaphorically and literally "fatally flawed." (Douard, 1990, p. 37)

Families affected by HIV must face the devastating diagnosis of a life-threatening disease and shoulder the burden of the stigma associated with that disease. It is the stigma of AIDS — whether the fear of retaliatory actions against those infected with the virus, or the feelings of worthlessness that infected people may have about themselves — that most often inhibits people from disclosing the diagnosis to others, including their own children. Families coping with AIDS are confronting stigma on both a societal and personal level on an almost daily basis.

Stigma and Discrimination: The AIDS Difference

AIDS is distinguished from other chronic or fatal illnesses because of the stigma associated with it. Stigma often leads to discrimination that, in its most extreme form, results in acts of rejection. In his landmark book, *The Nature of Prejudice*, Gordon Allport (1958) identified five types of rejective behavior [see box].

His 5-point scale distinguishes degrees of negative action, from relatively passive to the most aggressive.

Prejudice — A 5-Point Scale

1. **Antilocution** — Most people who have prejudices talk about them. They express their antagonism freely with like-minded friends, and occasionally with strangers. Many people do not go beyond this mild degree of antipathetic action.

2. **Avoidance** — If the prejudice is more intense, it leads the individual to avoid members of the disliked group, even at the cost of considerable inconvenience. In this case, the prejudiced person does not directly inflict harm upon the group he dislikes. He takes the burden of accommodation and withdrawal entirely upon himself.

3. **Discrimination** — Here the prejudiced person makes detrimental distinctions of an active sort. He undertakes to exclude all members of the group in question from certain types of employment, from residential housing, political rights, educational or recreational opportunities, churches, hospitals, or from some other social privileges. Segregation is an institutionalized form of discrimination, enforced legally or by common custom.

4. **Physical attack** — Under conditions of heightened emotion, prejudice may lead to acts of violence or semi-violence. An unwanted individual or family may be forcibly ejected from a neighborhood, or so severely threatened that they leave in fear.

5. **Extermination** — Lynchings, pogroms, massacres, and the Hitlerian program of genocide mark the ultimate degree of violent expression of prejudice.

Adapted from *The Nature Of Prejudice* by Gordon W. Allport, Doubleday Anchor Books, New York, 1958.

Examples of four types of rejective behavior have been reported by families since the beginning of the HIV epidemic. In Chapter I, Jennifer's description of the negative ways her family members talk among themselves about people with AIDS is an example of what Allport calls antilocution. Many parents describe the "avoidance" behavior of friends and family members who stop coming to visit their sick child once it becomes known the child is HIV infected. Examples of Allport's third category, discrimination, are plentiful; many children with AIDS, such as Ryan White, have been excluded from school, and refused admission to other community groups and activities. There are even examples of physical attacks against children and families — one has only to remember the Ray family in Florida whose home was burned. These examples of prejudice are frightening. It is no wonder that families guard the secret of AIDS so tightly.

Overcoming Societal Obstacles

A full discussion of the societal obstacles that force people to keep the secret of AIDS is beyond the scope of this book. Strategies that may be effective in overcoming these obstacles range from sweeping legislative actions and safeguards to the education of a single individual. This section will be limited to a discussion of two issues families say affect their decision to reveal their child's diagnosis. The first is the need for legislative safeguards that uphold and protect the rights of children with HIV infection to attend school; and the second is the need for accurate education for the community about pediatric HIV infection and the issues confronting children and their families.

The story of a noninfected sibling being barred from returning to his school once his sister's diagnosis became known was presented in Chapter I. It took a legal battle to have the child reinstated, and it was a much longer period of time before the infected sibling was able to gain entry into the school system. Since the beginning of the epidemic, this has been a controversial issue. It has divided communities, confounded educators, and ultimately resulted in tremendous pain for families and children with HIV/AIDS. Many families feel that if the educational system — a

social institution to which many look for enlightened leadership
— tolerates the stigmatization of infected children, there can be little hope that a less hostile atmosphere will prevail in society at
large. The importance of this issue is emphasized by a parent.

DORIS IS THE ADOPTIVE MOTHER of Keoke, age 9.
Keoke is aware of her diagnosis and participates in a
support group for HIV-infected children where she has the
opportunity to talk about her condition and treatment.
Doris has cared for Keoke since she was an infant, as well
as her twin sister Kerina, who is not infected. Doris talks
about how important the group is to Keoke, and expresses
her relief that this opportunity is open to the child. She
contrasts this with the "early days" when Keoke could not
gain readmission to school. At the age of 3, Keoke had been
placed in a class for preschool handicapped children due to
significant delays in her development. Once the local
school administrators became aware of her diagnosis,
Keoke was not allowed to participate in the classroom, nor
did she receive the services she needed. Doris became
involved in a landmark case to gain admittance to the
schools for HIV-infected children. She often talks of her
dismay and anger that the educational system should
make it so difficult for children.

Doris: "To me it seemed that if anything went down to
keep these kids segregated from the school system, they
would be segregated everywhere else in society. There was
already plenty of discrimination and all round bad
attitudes going on towards adults with AIDS, and I fought
this whenever I came across it.

"But I never expected that people would try and do the
same thing to children who cannot fight for themselves. So
I had to fight for Keoke, and hopefully, in helping her, I
would be helping other children and families. I had an
opportunity once, in the midst of all this fighting, to be on
a panel with a lot of teachers and other educators. I told
them they should be ashamed of themselves. I told them
they should be the ones on the front lines helping us to
overcome this stigma. I pointed out to them that next to the
parents, they were the ones who spent the most time with

children and should have their care and protection near to their hearts. I told them that if they didn't fight this prejudice and stigma, everything else would fail, and they would be condemning children and families living with AIDS to live in isolation and rejection."

The story of Doris and Keoke exemplifies the amazing capacity for leadership that many families living with HIV and AIDS have shown. Doris's persistence and determination to have what was right and just for her child has benefited all children with HIV in this country.

The following story of another parent's creative and tireless efforts to help educate the community in which she and her child live demonstrates the critical importance of education in the fight to end discrimination against children and families with HIV and AIDS.

FROM THE EARLIEST DAYS of learning her daughter's diagnosis, Joan, introduced in Chapter I, guarded the secret with fierce intensity. However, Joan often stated that the issue was not *if* the diagnosis would become known, but *when* it would. She felt strongly that the general climate in the nation at large, and in her own community, was still one of ignorance and fear. She stated, "I felt that until people got more educated, calmed down, I could not tell."

So Joan took it upon herself to participate in the education of her community, while still guarding the identity of her family. The following is Joan's story as related to the author over a period of months. It is, therefore, a necessarily condensed version of Joan's remarkable efforts, related in an effort to demonstrate the creative way one person sought to offer her unique personal experiences to educate her community.

Joan: "For the past few years I have been working with the County Health Department anonymously. I called them up and told them I was interested in working with them on education about HIV/AIDS. I gave them a false name, but I also told them this was not my real name. Nor did I tell them the city in which our family lived. I told them I was the mother of a child with HIV infection who was asymptomatic. They expressed a lot of interest in my situation. They told me there were other children in the county who were infected who were younger and sicker than my child. They also said that all of the children they had known had died when they were very young. They had not known any older, infected children who were healthy. It was clear they had a lot to learn about pediatric HIV infection and I felt I was in a unique position to supplement their education. In order that they could validate the truth of my story, I had made an arrangement ahead of time with my daughter's doctor, so that they could contact him and verify the story. The doctor knew the name I would be using in order to protect my family's true identity and he agreed to cooperate in the plan.

"After this was done, I began to meet with representatives from the County Health Department over a period of months. Initially, we met in a restaurant outside the area where I lived. So that they could contact me if they needed my help, my best friend, Pat, agreed to be the liaison between us.

"At this point I felt very strongly that education was the only thing we had to combat the fear, ignorance, and thus the stigma of AIDS, and I felt that I was in a better position than most to tell the Health Department the facts about pediatric HIV infection. Most of the information they had was based on the very few cases they had ever known. Since AIDS was the reportable end of the HIV spectrum of infection, they had never known a healthy child who was infected. Therefore, the information they had to use in educating the community was extremely limited. I was able to help them understand that one of the reasons they knew so little was because so many families, like my own, were in hiding. I was able to help them to see that although the mortality rate for AIDS is high, people are also *living* with HIV and AIDS."

While continuing to work with her County Health Department as a volunteer advisor and consultant, Joan began to reach out on the federal level. In the fall of 1990,

Joan experienced a period of depression and as she describes it, "when I get to the point of being upset or depressed, I turn around and do something drastic." Joan decided to approach her congressman in an effort to develop the kind of relationship with him that she now had with her County Health Department.

Joan: "When I called his office and related my story, the secretary asked me if I would consider speaking to the committee the congressman was involved with. This was the Select Committee on Children, Youth and Families. I told them I was interested, and once again my friend, Pat, agreed to act as the intermediary between the congressman's office and myself, thus continuing to protect my family's identity. This was in late September of 1990. Later in October, I was already planning to go to Washington to participate in the ACCH Family Network Meeting. The congressman assigned a staff member on the committee to arrange a meeting for me.

"I knew the congressman by reputation; he had always done a lot of work advocating for the rights of children with disabilities so I wasn't surprised at his interest. However, I was surprised at how quickly he responded to the story I had to tell. I was not using my real name and they knew that, so they could not use me for publicity purposes. It was clear he was acting out of a concern for the plight of children who are HIV infected and their families. During our meeting I made him aware of all the issues, and particularly stressed the need for education in the community at large. I told him that even if 95% of the community were behind me (supportive) it would be the 5% radical fringe that parents like myself have to fear. I talked to him about the need for more rights for foster parents of HIV-infected children. I was conscious that, even though I had acted out of my own particular and individual situation, I had a responsibility and an opportunity to be an advocate for all children and families infected and affected by HIV and AIDS. Although the congressman was extremely busy and the time originally scheduled for our meeting was very brief, he spent much more time than planned with me. He also sent an aide from

the staff of the Select Committee back to the ACCH
meeting with me so that other families could also share
their experiences with him."

Thus, Joan worked steadily over a period of years to educate
people at the local and national levels about the needs of children
and families affected by HIV. She continues to engage in these activities to this day.

It is important to note that as unique and inspired as Joan's
approach is in attempting to combat the stigma of AIDS through
education, her story is not an isolated one. So very many of the
families encountered by this author over the past six years have
struggled, whether anonymously or in the open, to advocate for
their children and families, and, indeed, for all families affected by
HIV and AIDS. In our efforts to combat the stigma of AIDS in
society at large — a stigma that forces so many people into hiding
— the stories of these valiant families stand out. Their words and
their experiences inspire us to join them in fighting the stigma and
ignorance that lead to discrimination against families struggling
with HIV and AIDS.

Coming to Terms With Stigma as a Personal Struggle

In addition to the external manifestations of stigmatization,
such as exclusion from school, people belonging to stigmatized
groups must also struggle with internal conflicts and doubts. It
has been noted that members of stigmatized groups often have
very negative feelings about themselves (Goffman, 1963). It is a
sad reality that many family members affected by HIV hold the
same beliefs and feelings about themselves that are held about
them by nonstigmatized people in society at large.

For those who work with or care about families affected by
HIV, it is essential to understand the debilitating impact of being a
stigmatized person, as well as to develop some strategies that can
be used to counteract this potentially immobilizing factor. Unless
a parent has had the opportunity to explore and come to terms
with the meaning of the AIDS-stigma association in her own

mind, it is unlikely that she will consider disclosing the diagnosis to anyone — especially a child.

In Chapter I, parents said they believed their children thought that AIDS only happened to bad people. Yet many parents reveal that they, too, hold this view. This is often expressed as punishment by God for wrongdoing. Consider the statements of two HIV-infected women upon learning their child's diagnosis.

> *Transfusion recipient:* "I used to laugh at Jehovah's Witnesses because they didn't believe in blood transfusions. Maybe God is punishing me for laughing at someone else's religious beliefs."

> *Former IV drug user:* "I'm an addict, but I had been clean for two years when my baby was born. I guess God must have felt I had to be punished for all the harm I did."

These feelings of guilt may be one of the central influences on parents' unwillingness to reveal the diagnosis, as illustrated in the following story.

> CLAIRE IS THE MOTHER of 10-month-old Kate. Claire and her husband Alan live in the same household as Claire's parents. Claire and her husband are both HIV positive and asymptomatic, although Claire has some minor dermatological problems. Kate has AIDS and has been admitted to the hospital because of severe infections. Claire has refused to allow her parents to visit the infant; she has not revealed Kate's true diagnosis to them and fears they might accidentally learn it if they come to the hospital to visit.

> Claire initially told her parents that Kate has a rare form of leukemia and that the doctors have advised that only parents are allowed to visit in order to diminish the risk of outside infections. At first, Claire's father accepts these terms, but his probing questions about Kate's "leukemia" become more and more difficult for Claire to answer, and she talks about the stress this is causing her. When asked by a social worker to consider whether the stress of keeping the secret may not be greater than the risk of

telling her father the real diagnosis, Claire answers in the following way.

Claire: "Nothing could be worse than telling him the truth. You cannot imagine what will happen if I do that. You see, he never wanted me to marry Alan in the first place. He never really got along with him. He used to tell me that my life would come to a bad end if Alan and I got married. He didn't even know that Alan used drugs in the past, yet he really disliked him. Imagine if he had known that Alan was a drug user and through his drug use had become infected. Then Alan infected me, and I infected the baby. I was raised to be very religious and to obey the Ten Commandments. The Commandments say 'honor thy father and thy mother,' but I disobeyed my father's wishes and married Alan. Now what he said has come true. My life is coming to a bad end. I disobeyed my father, which means I disobeyed God's Commandments. Now God is punishing me for being a bad person."

Claire often spoke of the shame and guilt she felt for "what she had done," and also said that she experienced these feelings more strongly when in the presence of her parents.

Another parent of an HIV-infected child talked about the self-hatred she was experiencing, and described an incident that occurred in the course of doing her housework.

Parent: "I was washing dishes this morning, and I felt so down. I knew that my daughter would be having a spinal tap today, and I knew how much it would hurt her. As I completed cleaning the sink, I found myself staring at the scummy residue in the bottom of the sink, and all of a sudden I realized I was saying to myself, 'That's just what you are, scum! You did this to your baby.'"

Parents may also be unsure of how others feel, even when they are apparently accepting.

Parent: "My mother knows that my son has AIDS and she has always been very supportive of my husband and me. Often she takes care of my son so that I can run errands or go to my doctor's. Even so, I never feel certain of how she really feels. Last week I asked her to babysit so I could go and get my hair done. She said she couldn't do it because she had a cold and didn't want to pass it on to the baby. I found myself doubting her word. I wondered if she was angry with me because the baby is infected. Then I told myself that maybe she really is afraid she can catch the virus from the baby."

This same mother went on to discuss how frequently these moments of feeling unsure arose for her, which in turn led to renewed feelings of shame and guilt for the fact that she had passed the virus on to her child. Whenever her best friend pointed out that it was not her fault since she had not known she was infected, she responded:

> *Parent:* "Well you might think that, but I have been reading a lot about women who are infected and then they get pregnant. I found out that not every baby who is born to a woman who is infected gets the virus. So why did I give it to my baby? Well, there must have been something wrong with me, maybe I was too defective to have a baby in the first place. I probably should have had my tubes tied so I could never have a baby. If my baby dies, I am the one responsible."

The feeling by this mother that "something must have been wrong with me" has been shared by other parents and family members.

> DARLEEN IS THE MOTHER of Pat, a 31-year-old woman who is an active IV drug user. Darleen is the legal guardian of her grandchildren, Pat's children, Rhonda and Al-Karim. Both Pat and Rhonda have AIDS. Al-Karim is uninfected. Rhonda has been in the hospital for a long period of time due to multiple AIDS-related infections and illnesses. She experiences a great deal of pain much of the time, and her physical pain is reflected in the tremendous emotional pain that Darleen experiences as she sits for many hours by the child's bedside. One day, Darleen

overhears a conversation at the nearby nurse's station, and she discusses it with the social worker:

Darleen: "I heard them talking about the mother of another child who has AIDS. This parent gives them a lot of trouble, she is very aggressive, constantly complaining, and also she comes to the hospital when she is high and this makes them very angry. When they were talking about her, they were saying that they thought she was so aggressive because she was really feeling guilty at being responsible for her child's condition. One of the nurses, who is very close to this mother, said the mother had said 'if my child dies I will have become a murderer.' The nurses were very upset that the mother felt this way about herself. As I listened to them talking, I was thinking 'how do they think I feel.' If Pat and Rhonda die, I will have been responsible for two deaths. I brought Pat into this world and she became a drug addict. Then she had Rhonda, and now they both have AIDS. Whichever way I look at it, I keep finding that there must be something wrong with me for this to be happening, since it all started with me."

Goffman (1963) has stated that stigma spoils the social identity of a person and "has the effect of cutting him off from society and from himself, so that he stands a discredited person facing an unaccepting world" (p. 19). This isolation, with its attendent feelings of guilt, shame, and self-doubt contributes to the reluctance of family members to share the diagnosis with others. When those infected and most intimately affected have internalized negative attitudes about themselves, it is very unlikely that they will reveal their situation to anyone. Their intense self-hatred makes them feel unworthy to receive comfort and support from friends, family, or even the professional community.

Coping With Feelings of Shame and Guilt

Guilt and shame are among the most devastating feelings experienced by stigmatized people. In her book, *Coping with Stigma*, McFarland (1989) describes these feelings this way:

Shame is the painful feeling arising from the consciousness of something dishonorable, improper, or ridiculous done by oneself or another. It is a feeling about oneself as a person. Guilt is a feeling of responsibility or remorse for some real or imagined offense or crime. Put more simply, shame is about who you are, or believe yourself to be; guilt is about what you do or believe you did that was harmful or wrong. (p. 82)

Parents who are HIV infected often devalue themselves by listening to what McFarland refers to as the "inner voice of shame." This voice tells the parent that she is not worthy, and hinders her ability to care for her child, and especially to care for herself. Feelings of unworthiness lead parents to neglect their own health and refuse medical treatment — a familiar phenomenon among families affected by HIV.

Professionals can help parents become aware of these inner voices of shame, doubt, and despair that erode their sense of competence and self-esteem. In an earlier example, the mother who referred to herself as scum was listening to her inner voice of shame. Her social worker suggested that she reflect back to the moment she described herself this way to see if there was an inner voice at work. Upon reflection, the parent became aware that she often felt there was an ugly monster inside of her trying to pull her down.

> *Social worker:* "You have said you do recognize that there is a kind of inner voice speaking, and you have described it like an ugly monster trying to pull you down. Where did this monster come from?"

> *Parent:* "Oh! I recognize this voice all right, it's from the time when I was using (drugs). I used to hear it quite a lot in those days, and it got so loud telling me what a low-life I was, that I would just go and do more drugs to drown it out."

> *Social worker:* "But now you are clean, and yet the ugly voice is still with you?"

> *Parent:* "Yes, I guess it is. I never really thought of it that way before. I left the drugs behind, and brought the monster with me."

After some period of time, this mother began to recognize that the ugly voice which "is like a monster pulling me down," is the voice of shame and guilt, and she recognized that she had not forgiven herself for her drug-using days. Some weeks later, she raised the topic with the social worker again, reporting that she had begun to explore the issue of self-forgiveness with her counselor at the drug treatment program. She described some of the insight she had gained.

> *Parent:* "I have been talking to my counselor about this voice thing, and she helped me to see it in another way. She said that as long as I allowed this voice to take control of my thoughts and feelings, I would be dragged down. She suggested it was as if I was allowing the old me (the drug user) to live on instead of the new me. When she said this, it was like a light bulb went on in my head, and I suddenly realized what she meant. It was a very hard struggle giving up drugs, but I didn't want my child to have a drug user for a mother, so when I became pregnant, I started to clean up my life. Thank God she came into the world drug-free, and I am very proud of that. I think I have done a very good job with her. I have good friends, and my family and I have been reunited. I am not the person I used to be and I can't let that voice tell me I am."

Once the parent becomes aware of the inner voice, the possibility of sharing these destructive "messages" is opened up. Feelings of shame keep their power when they remain hidden and secret; sharing the feelings offers the prospect of easing the burden.

Professionals can also help parents increase their self-acceptance. To be self-accepting does not mean liking everything about oneself. It only means acknowledging something is true without imposing a judgment. The parent who has used drugs often feels guilty for infecting her child. To point out that it was a virus that led to AIDS may reflect the facts of the situation, but does not speak to the pain of the guilt feelings being communicated by the parent. In the presence of a compassionate, empathic, and caring professional, the parent may have the opportunity to ventilate over and over again these painful feelings in the security of a nonjudgmental environment. This cathartic experience often deepens the parent/professional relationship so that new hope can be found. In learning to let go of the past and live for the possibilities inherent in each day, the parent comes to see what is possible in the here and now that can enhance her self-esteem. Consider the following example.

> CALLIE IS THE MOTHER of 4-year-old Tashia, who is hospitalized for chronic upper-respiratory infection secondary to HIV infection. Callie is a former drug user and prostitute. She is a conscientious and tender parent to Tashia and is skillful in helping Tashia withstand the rigors of frequent blood-drawing. She has a repertoire of skills which range from assuring, encouraging, and timely comforting, to the ability to distract her daughter with humor and song. Despite her enviable parental strengths, as her daughter's condition deteriorates, Callie is overwhelmed by feelings of guilt and shame, which she has begun to share with her social worker. Day after day, Callie refers to her past life and identifies herself as the cause of her daughter's predicament. Like many parents, she feels that she is being punished by God for past sins.

> Callie uses part of each visit with the social worker to give vent to these feelings that she has kept hidden for so long. Interjections by the social worker are offered only occasionally in an effort to counteract Callie's self-derogatory statements. When Callie states that she is no good, the social worker responds by saying that she understands Callie has terrible feelings about her past life and drug-using activity, but that it is clear from the love she shows her daughter that there was never an intent to do harm. The social worker then invites Callie to really gaze upon her daughter's face and see the love and trust Tashia holds for her mother. Tearfully, Callie affirms that it is true; whatever her past life has been, she is confident that she has been the best possible mother to Tashia.

> In time Callie's self-anger abates and she becomes better able to focus on who she knows she is *today* — a woman of strength and depth who is loved and trusted by her

daughter and admired and respected by others. Even more importantly, Callie declares that she will strive to make sure that the regrets she feels about the past will not rob her of the opportunity to live each day to the fullest.

The role of peer support

Finding comfort and support from sympathetic others enables people in stigmatized groups to cope with their situation (Goffman, 1963). In addition to receiving support from empathic professionals, members of stigmatized groups also find solace and strength among those who are similarly stigmatized. Families affected by HIV often remark on the sense of relief and release they

---

Ways in which stigmatized persons can learn to cope.

1. Become conscious of the inner voice of shame that carries self-derogatory messages.
2. Replace negative thoughts with positive thoughts.
3. Share the inner voice of shame with someone you trust.
4. Understand that self-acceptance does not mean liking everything about oneself. It means acknowledging something is true about oneself without judgment.
5. Become more nonjudgmental, able to look at one's own strengths and weaknesses. When the inner voice of shame points out faults or limitations, counteract this by naming a strength.
6. Learn to accept limitations and even weaknesses. It is much easier to change an undesired quality when not self-condemning.
7. Learn to live one day at a time.

Source: McFarland, R. (1989), *Coping With Stigma.* New York: The Rosen Publishing Group.

---

experience when meeting other families in the same situation. One mother stated that the anxiety she initially felt in bringing her child to the clinic for treatment was offset by her eagerness to sit with other mothers and openly discuss her situation, as well as her feelings, in a place where she would not have to look over her shoulder before saying the word AIDS.

Another parent described her loneliness when she first learned the diagnosis, and the relief she felt when she joined a parent support group.

> *Allisa:* "When I first started out with this I was alone on that mountaintop — feeling alone and isolated. I felt I was the only one on that mountaintop. Then I went to group and found I wasn't alone. I found there were many different kinds of parents in the group. Some had more money than me, and some had less than me; but regardless of where we came from, we all had these feelings, we all felt alone and afraid and outcast from the world. We all worried about the effect this would have on our families. You could be a rich white woman, or a working woman, or a woman who was a drug addict, but you were all feeling the same feelings and this was what we had in common."

This support group diminished Allisa's feelings of loneliness that resulted from the stigma and isolation of AIDS. In the company of other people sharing the same stigmatizing situation, she was able to talk about the diagnosis and its implications over and over again. Through the empathy and mutual compassion of such a support group, parents can regain self-esteem and hope. The peer support experience can also prepare the way for the possibility of disclosing the diagnosis outside the empathic circle.

Chapter Summary

There is a powerful stigma associated with the diagnosis of HIV and families affected by it are vulnerable to overt and covert acts of discrimination. Further, people with HIV often internalize society's negative attitudes and beliefs, leading to intense feelings of worthlessness. Professionals can play a valuable part in helping parents recognize the degree to which they have internalized these negative images, and assist them in replacing self-denigrating inner messages with more positive ones. Feelings of isolation and loneliness can also be reduced by participating in family-to-family support groups.

It is often in the company of caring professionals that parents first have the opportunity to discuss the diagnosis and its impact on them. However, it is in communion with other families facing the challenges of AIDS that parents are most free to discuss the diagnosis and its implications again and again. This experience is invaluable for parents as they move towards revealing the diagnosis to other adults, and also to their children.

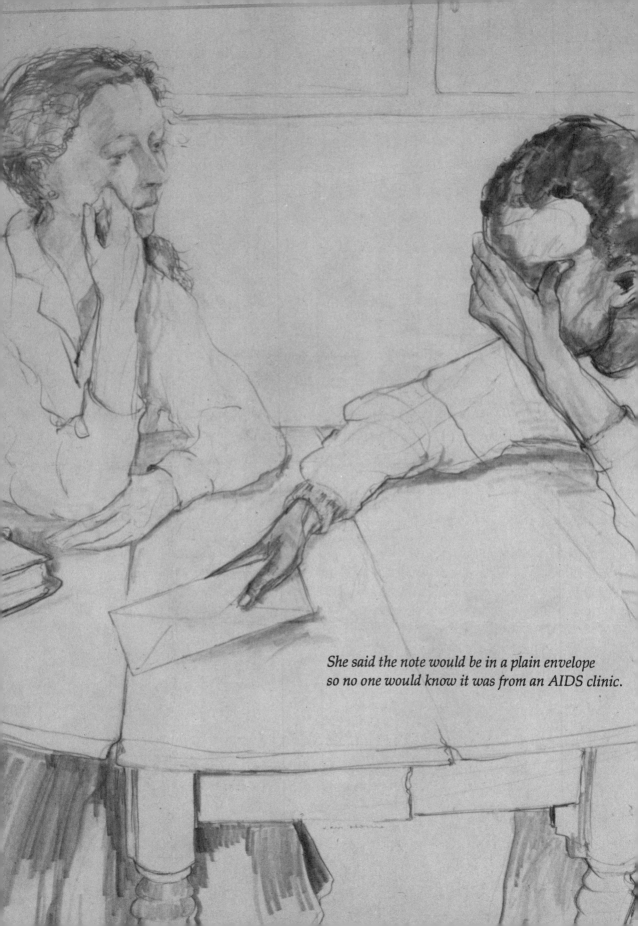

She said the note would be in a plain envelope so no one would know it was from an AIDS clinic.

CHAPTER IV

The Four Phases of Disclosure

In 1969, in her book *On Death and Dying*, Elisabeth Kubler-Ross attempted to summarize what she had learned from patients facing terminal illness. She proposed a series of stages through which individuals progress as they come to terms with their illness. Kubler-Ross's work has provided a framework for understanding the feelings and concerns of people with terminal illness. However, there is a danger in over-simplifying the concepts she presents. In attempting to categorize people in stages, it is easy to deny individual realities and the dynamic nature of human experience. Nevertheless, Kubler-Ross's stages have proved invaluable in reflecting the perspectives and coping mechanisms of dying people and their families.

It is with these thoughts in mind — the value of categorizing experiences, balanced by the risks involved in stereotyping a particular family's experience — that the idea of phases of disclosure is proposed. These phases are purely the conceptualization of the author. They may be thought of as points along a continuum — with secrecy about the diagnosis, on one end, to full disclosure of the diagnosis on the other. Neither end of this continuum is "better" or more advanced than the other. This conceptualization of phases does not suggest that all families automatically start at the secrecy stage, and progress to disclosure. However, the proposed stages are useful in describing the experiences and challenges families face at different points in time.

Secrecy Phase

Characteristics of the secrecy phase

A parent has learned the diagnosis of HIV/AIDS for the first time. The infected person may be herself, her child, or another family member. She is in a state of shock and anguish, facing the possibility of the death of one or more members of the family. Vows are made not to disclose the diagnosis to anyone, adult or child. The parent is in a state of extreme isolation and loneliness, despite an outward appearance of normalcy.

The professional at the clinic or hospital may be the only person with whom the parent can experience some sense of release and relief by discussing the diagnosis, as well as fears that the secret may be discovered. In this phase the parent tells the child little, if anything, about the diagnosis or the reasons for clinic visits or hospitalizations. On a practical level, it is easier to maintain the secret if the infected person is asymptomatic. Some parents who are HIV positive have talked about arranging their clinic visits to coincide with the child's school hours. In cases where children are HIV infected but well, their clinic visits may seem no different than the experience of any child visiting his pediatrician or clinic for a regular check-up.

At this stage, the adult who is aware of the diagnosis is coping not only with the traumatic news, but also with the strain of living with the secret.

Parent/professional relationship in the secrecy phase

Parents seek reassurance that professionals respect their confidentiality and support them in their decision. A parent may seek this reassurance repeatedly over an extended period of time. The willingness of professionals to anticipate and offer this support will provide great comfort to the parent.

> *Father:* "After I got over the first shock of knowing that my wife, son, and I were HIV infected, I was terrified that anyone would find out. Mostly I was afraid that if the landlord discovered, he might try to evict us from the

apartment. The nurse at the clinic seemed to understand my feelings without my telling her. She told me she would send me a note to confirm my son's next clinic appointment. She also said that the note would be sent in a plain envelope so no one would know it was from an AIDS clinic. This made me feel relieved. She understood how afraid I was someone might accidentally find out. I knew it would be much easier to talk to her about other concerns I had, and that she would understand and care about my family."

When the parent feels confident that his wish to maintain secrecy is anticipated, understood, accepted, and respected, there is an increased likelihood that he will be able to talk with the professional about the implications of keeping the secret. The professional can create a trusting and safe environment for the parent by asking about stresses entailed in maintaining secrecy. Such inquiries deepen the trust that parents hold for professionals.

Mother: "The last time I visited the clinic I met with my child's social worker. She knows I haven't even told my twin sister that my baby and I have the virus, and she asked me how it is for me when my sister comes to visit my house. I burst into tears and told her that my sister's visits create a lot of tension since I have to be careful I won't make a slip and talk about the clinic. This is extremely difficult for me since my sister and I have always told each other everything. I just can't tell her now, but I feel like I'm cheating our relationship in not telling her. The social worker understood and said it must be very painful for me to keep the secret. She asked me what I imagined my sister might do if I did tell her. I told her that deep in my heart I felt my sister would stand by me, even if she was devastated at first. I was surprised when I realized how I had answered the social worker's question, because all I had been looking at was how I would feel if my sister rejected me. I also really appreciated the fact that the social worker was concentrating on *my* feelings about keeping the secret. I knew *she* felt it might be easier if I told my sister, so I was happy to know that she didn't use the occasion to try and get me to tell my sister."

This story raises an important point. While it is recognized that the parent should be at the center of the decision-making process, especially on the issue of disclosing the diagnosis to children, this does not mean that the professional cannot contribute to the discussion. Many professionals do hold strong beliefs that it is better for the child to know the diagnosis. To pretend indifference about whether the child knows the diagnosis or not is dishonest and it is inevitable that the parent will sense the deception. This, in turn, may lead to parents withholding *their* true feelings about the issue and avoiding any discussion.

Professionals often attempt to conceal their feelings about a parent's decision, especially if they feel the decision is unwise. They may do this in an effort to keep the relationship on a pleasant, noncontroversial basis. Keith-Lucas (1972) insists that "the attempt to keep the relationship on a pleasant level is the greatest source of ineffectual helping known to people" (p. 18).

The parent/professional relationship is precisely that, a relationship. There is a need for openness and honesty on both sides. The parent anticipates that the professional may have a different point of view; consideration of another perspective can be helpful to the parent in decision making. It is a patent untruth that the parent wishes only for a mirror in the relationship when difficult decisions are being weighed. Rather, professionals should offer the parent a window of other views, for a window sheds light.

Parent-to-parent (or other adult) relationship in the secrecy phase

Some parents in this phase choose a professional with whom to discuss their feelings. Others may also identify another adult to whom they can disclose the diagnosis and gain relief from the agonizing burden of being alone with the secret.

> *Eva:* "I had decided that only the immediate members of my family needed to know about my daughter and granddaughter. I didn't want my family to experience any discrimination or reprisals — the kind of thing you hear about all the time, people losing jobs and their homes being

burned down. So for quite a while only the immediate family knew. In many ways they needed to lean on me. So I decided I would have to be the strong one to help everyone keep it together. Still, there were times when I felt *I* needed a friend and I began to think about this a lot. As I looked around at all the people I knew outside the family, I tried to figure out if this or that one would be someone I could tell. I began to listen closely to their attitudes about other people, particularly if they talked about people with AIDS. I think I was weighing up the risks, and deciding who might be safe to tell. Who did I know who was not a gossip, could keep a confidence, was compassionate and cared about me and mine? I suppose it was a question of values.

"At this time, there was a member of my church, Essie, and she and I became quite close. She lived with a lot of her family members, and there were some problems with alcoholism in the family. Life was often very tough for Essie, and she and I used to talk for long periods of time on the phone. She and I are deeply rooted in our religion, and there were so many times when I felt we were on the exact same wavelength. One day we were talking on the phone and she asked me to say some prayers for her and her family. That's when I decided to take that chance and reach out to her. I told her my daughter and granddaughter had the virus. It just came out naturally because of the type of spirit that existed between us at that time.

"In my church there is a saying 'try the spirit, by the spirit,' and this saying has a lot of meaning for me. It refers to how genuine you are in your spiritual beliefs. In my church, especially on a Sunday, there is a lot of preaching and singing, clapping and dancing, and calling out. This is how it can be when you are moved with the spirit. But there are a lot of people who shout and wail and it is all a show. They wear their religious convictions and discard them as easily as they put on and take off their Sunday clothes. The minister cautions about this sort of thing all the time. The spirit is how you live your whole life, not how loud you pray.

"I feel Essie is this kind of person and I sensed it was right to tell her. The instant I told her, my load already felt lighter. She told me she was so sorry and promised she would pray for me and my family. She said she would stay with me: 'Sister, we will pray together on this and just take it one day at a time.'

"There is a great comfort once you know you will not have to face this whole burden alone. It still hurts and there is a lot of pain, but the load gets considerably easier when it is shared. Once I had Essie to talk to, it made keeping the secret a much easier task. I have to say another thing about Essie, and how I know now that my instinct to tell her back then was the true instinct, guided by the spirit. When my daughter got sick and had to be hospitalized I still had to go to work. Even though I would spend every evening with her, that still meant a lot of time when she would be alone. Essie would go up there and visit her for hours on end, bringing her food and little presents, even though Essie had very little money. It was a great comfort to me that my daughter was not alone. But the biggest-hearted, most compassionate thing Essie ever did was at my daughter's funeral. When it came time for them to close the lid to the casket, Essie stood in front of me so I would not see the light closed out for the last time on my daughter's face."

Exploratory Phase

Characteristics of the exploratory phase

Although parents continue to maintain secrecy about the HIV diagnosis, the intensity with which they guard, and are consumed by, the secret lessens over time.

Having gained some relief from the isolation of keeping the secret through a one-on-one relationship with a professional, family member, or friend, parents may be interested in discussing the issues and feelings with a wider group, such as a parent support group. In the secrecy phase, parents may have been reluctant to join a group for fear of encountering someone from their neighborhood or circle of friends. In the exploratory phase they realize that even if they do encounter someone they know, that person will also be concerned about maintaining confidentiality.

Additionally, parents in this phase may begin to show some ambivalence about keeping the secret from the child, while still asserting that it is better for the child not to be told. Although parents may not be willing to give the name HIV or AIDS to the diagnosis, they may feel ready to offer some explanation to the child, using euphemisms, or accurate descriptions of HIV/AIDS short of saying the actual words. Certainly, in this phase, parents of HIV-infected children display increased interest in talking to their children about the treatment regimen and clinic procedures, and are more conscious of helping them cope with stressful medical events and hospitalizations.

Parent/professional relationship in the exploratory phase

Professionals who are attentive to the manifestations of the ambivalence in this phase may open up the topic with parents and explore whether they are moving toward disclosure.

> *Professional:* "Melody was 6 years old when she was first diagnosed, and her mother always insisted that she would never dream of disclosing the diagnosis to her. In the beginning when she brought Melody to the clinic, she was clearly terrified that someone would mention AIDS in Melody's presence and she would frequently seek reassurance that everyone would keep the secret. When she noticed Melody talking to another child, she would whisk her away immediately, fearful the other child might know more than Melody did. Now Melody is 7, and I noticed a change coming over her mother. She allows Melody to play with other children and no longer shoos her from the room when the doctor comes in to talk. One day I asked her if she had changed her mind about Melody finding out the diagnosis, and she declared that she had not. I then pointed out the changes I had noticed, and after reflecting on my observation for a while, she smiled and said that maybe she was not as nervous as she used to be about Melody finding out. Although overall she wished that Melody

didn't have to know, she stated that sooner or later she guessed that Melody would be ready."

At this stage, the parent shows increasing concern about the infected child's anxiety in coming to the clinic or undergoing painful procedures. In this phase the parent will value collaborating with the professional on ways to help the child manage these stressful experiences.

> JOEL WAS ABOUT TO participate in a clinical trial for AZT, and an appointment has been scheduled for several tests, including a lumbar puncture (spinal tap). His parents met with the social worker at the clinic to discuss Joel's fears about the procedure, as well as their own anxieties in helping Joel through the procedure.
>
> *Andrew:* "My problem is that I cannot even be here on the day he is to have the tap done. In a way I'm relieved, but I also feel guilty about not being here to help Joel and support Simone."
>
> *Simone:* "I would just like to find some more ways to discuss this with Joel — to help him feel less anxious about it. Even though I'm going to be in the room with Joel when they are doing the tap, I'm afraid I might fall apart when he needs me."

The social worker discussed the issue in detail with Andrew and Simone and the three of them then met with a nurse from the team to go over what they could expect during the procedure. The social worker also gave the parents a book about children with cancer undergoing a spinal tap. Relevant pages from the book were copied, and Andrew and Simone used them to go over the procedure with Joel. Additionally, the social worker agreed to be available on the day of the procedure to provide support and encouragement to Simone and Joel if they should need it.

On the day the spinal tap was to be performed, Joel arrived at the clinic much more confident than before, and said he had learned several ways to "get through it." The social worker, on request, was present with the family as the procedure was being performed, and, together with Simone, Joel, and the nurse, sang a song that Joel had rehearsed with his parents as a way to get through the painful part of the procedure. Afterwards, Simone and Joel laughed and made jokes about how crazy it would have looked to an outsider to see us all singing "old MacDonald had a farm" while, as Joel put it, "the doctor was shoving a giant needle in my spine."

Parent-to-parent (or other adult) relationship in the exploratory phase

Having had some period of time in which to talk about the diagnosis with a small number of trusted relatives or friends, a parent who was initially reluctant to join a support group may now wish to meet other parents who share her experience. In the previous chapter, Allisa talked about the decrease in isolation she experienced when she first joined a parent support group. Later when Allisa's anxiety about guarding the secret of AIDS was lessened, she began to use her support group to explore the possibility of disclosing the diagnosis to her daughter.

Allisa: "I began to realize that the support group I was involved with was a good place to discuss the different feelings I had about telling my daughter the diagnosis. In the beginning I was very clear that I did not want to tell her the diagnosis, but as time went by, sometimes I would begin to think about telling her. As I went through these changes, I was able to talk out all my feelings and thoughts with my group. When I would consider the possibility of telling my daughter, I would discuss things like what words to use, and the group would give me feedback. By this I do not mean that I accepted all the advice I was given, but just by getting a lot of different thoughts and ideas from families in the same situation as myself, it helped me to clear up my thoughts.

"Being with other parents who are in your same situation, and therefore can *really* understand what you are experiencing is such a relief. You can talk about anything and know that there are others who understand because they have been through or are going through the same things. It helps you to not feel so alone and scared. You get courage through it and it helps you to plan your next moves and to make your mind up about how you want to handle things, especially about telling your child the diagnosis."

Readiness Phase

Characteristics of the readiness phase

In this phase parents move closer to revealing the diagnosis to the child. They begin to activate plans for disclosure. Often, though by no means always, parents may enlist the cooperation of a trusted professional as they move toward disclosure.

Parent/professional relationship in the readiness phase

ALLISA HAS MOVED closer to the point of revealing to Keesha that she is HIV infected, although she is still not ready to say the word AIDS. Allisa has given her consent for Keesha to participate in a support group for HIV-infected children. The group is facilitated by the social worker who is on the health team following Keesha and other children who are involved in a study of children receiving AZT. The purpose of the group is to give children an opportunity to talk about issues related to their treatment regimen. Some children in the group have been told the diagnosis by their parents, others have not. Allisa develops a plan with the social worker, Janie, before allowing Keesha to join the group.

Allisa: "I have given Janie the green light. If Keesha asks her any questions, she can answer them honestly. Also, whenever Keesha and I have discussions about her illness or her clinic visits, I let Janie know what we discussed so that she and I can respond to Keesha along the same lines. Janie knows that I do not want her to say HIV or AIDS to Keesha. Right now, Keesha has just been told that she has a virus in her blood and that is why she has to take the medicine. I have set up a plan with Janie if Keesha should ever ask about AIDS. Janie will tell Keesha, 'Oh, I see you are thinking about AIDS. Let me talk to Mommy and then we will all talk some more about it together.' That way Keesha will know she is not being ignored, but Janie and I will have a chance to talk about it before I decide what to do next."

In this way, Allisa was able to use the trusting relationship she had developed with her child's social worker to gradually move toward disclosure. This same relationship is described from the social worker's perspective.

Janie: "We suggested to the parents that we bring the children together to share their experiences. While some children had been told their diagnosis, other parents were adamant that the child should not be told. I made it very clear that I absolutely respected their right of decision making, and that I would not tell their children the diagnosis. However, I also made it clear that when children asked questions I would let them fully explore their own questions and not try to change the subject. I also told the parents that I felt that many of the children might be aware of things we adults feel they don't know. The parents were willing to have me talk about 'a germ in the blood' or about 'kids who have to go to the hospital.' When I asked them if I could talk about having a virus, they said it was okay as long as I didn't say AIDS."

Several months after Keesha joined the group a teacher at her school saw her taking her medicine and asked her if it was AZT. Keesha went home and asked her mother for the first time what the name of the virus was. Her mother was stunned.

Allisa: "Keesha came home from school that day and told me a teacher had seen her taking her medicine, and had asked her if it was AZT. Keesha told the teacher she didn't know, but she then asked me, 'What medicine am I taking?' By this time, I had promised myself that I wouldn't lie to her any more, so when she asked me if she was taking AZT, I told her she was. She asked me, 'What is wrong with me?' It was such a shock when she asked me this. I was not prepared for it. I did not want to say AIDS and I still don't want to say it. I also told her that this was personal information, and it is not the school's business or the street's business. I told her she could talk to Janie about it. Then I called Janie and told her I wanted to speak with her about what Keesha and I had discussed."

Janie: "Allisa pulled me aside prior to the beginning of the group and told me what had happened between her and Keesha. She told me that when Keesha had asked her the name of the virus, she said she'd forgotten the name. Allisa and I then began to brainstorm how we could respond. I showed Allisa a book I had called *Jimmy and the Eggs Virus* (a book about a little boy who discovers, accidentally, he has AIDS) and asked if she thought we should read the book to the children. She said, 'Maybe it's time.' I told her I would have to ask permission of the other parents before reading it in the group. However, I suggested that until then I could lead the group in a discussion about the topic of private information. Allisa was enthusiastic and this is what I did.

"I presented a scenario to the children of a mommy and daddy who had a big argument and asked the children to discuss their ideas about whom the children could tell. This helped us to move to a more general discussion on the kinds of information that are public and the kinds that are private. The discussion helped the children clarify differences between public and private information and identify when and with whom certain information could be shared. This set the stage for a later discussion about the AIDS diagnosis, and the need to keep the information private."

Keesha's story provides an excellent example of parent/professional collaboration. Both parties respect the skills and knowledge of the other. While the parent is clearly in charge of decision making, the professional's perspective is highly valued. The parent is quite clear about where she wants to go, but turns to a professional she trusts and respects to help her reach her destination.

Parent-to-parent (or other adult)
relationship at the readiness phase

Parents may seek the help of a professional to discuss the possibility of disclosing the diagnosis to their child, or they may discuss it with another trusted adult. Dana states that as she moved closer to revealing the diagnosis to her children, she began sharing the diagnosis with more people in her adult circle.

> *Dana:* "It was as if I was saying to myself, 'Okay, so you have told your family now, but they *should* be supportive, how is the rest of the world going to be?' If my children were going to know, even though I might urge them to keep it secret, I realized they could let it slip. So I think I was trying to test out the attitudes of other adults to AIDS. Maybe if negative reactions happened there, I would re-think my decision to tell my children. So I began looking for clues if I could tell other people, and who they would be. I remember once after some of us had attended a seminar on AIDS and women, we had returned to work and were doing some role-plays. I suddenly decided to do some instant role-play without telling the rest of the staff what I was doing, so I said, 'Well I have something to tell you all, I am HIV infected.' I felt sure that one staff member pulled back from me as I said this, and I know everyone was shocked and reacted in some way. Now, looking back I realize this was a foolish thing to do and anyone would have reacted under the circumstances, but I also remember it making a big impression on me. Mostly I was sorry I had done it. Of course, I told them all I was just doing a role-play and everyone relaxed. But the most important thing I remember was that the social worker was the only one who didn't react strongly. She just looked up from her work, looked into my eyes kind of sadly, and then, when I said I had been role-playing, looked me right in the eye again, smiled a little, and went quietly back to work. At that moment, I knew I was going to end up telling her.

> "She and I had started to be a little friendly, and we sometimes went out to lunch together, or occasionally to a movie at night. We were becoming friends. She was telling me some things about her life and I was telling her about mine. I began to drop hints that I had a very big situation

in my life that I wasn't telling too many people about and saying that I was trying to decide how to talk to my children about it. One day when we went out for a ride, I told her how much I was enjoying getting to know her, and how much I appreciated different times when she had supported and comforted me at work when I felt down. We started to talk about how stress can affect your work and how you cannot tell everyone your problems. We started to tell each other more personal things about ourselves and she told me some painful experiences she had in the past. I remember us both saying how good it was when you could find someone to trust and confide in. That's when I decided it was time to plunge in and take a risk. I asked her what she would say if I told her I was HIV infected. She said to me, 'I think I would feel very sad for you. Is that what you *are* telling me now?' I said that it was, and commented that she didn't seem so shocked. She told me that she had felt for some time that I wanted to tell her whatever my 'big situation' was, and she said she guessed it must be something very personal and difficult to tell. She said that she had just waited for me to be ready to tell if and when I wanted to.

"I know it was this incident that helped me move ahead and get ready to tell the children. This was something she and I talked about a lot. How do you tell your children something like this? She had a teenage daughter so she and I had a lot in common talking about how you raise teenagers, and how you talk to them about the hard stuff, stuff your mother never talked to you about. I asked her if she thought I should tell Alicia and Omar, but she said that I knew she couldn't tell me what decision to make. I laughed when she said, 'You know you and I don't really take advice from anyone, and that is one of the problems we have in common.' She added, 'I think you have already made up your mind to tell them, and it's just a case of when.' She was right about that, too!"

Disclosure Phase

Over time, some parents will decide to tell their child the diagnosis. Some will simply choose what they feel is the most appropriate time and tell the child in their own home without consulting a professional. Others having decided to disclose, seek the input and assistance of a trusted professional. Together, the parent and professional can weigh how, where, and with whom the discussion of the diagnosis should occur. Consideration should be given to the child's age and developmental level as well as the words that will be used. Role-playing the actual disclosure can help parents anticipate their child's reactions or questions and practice their responses. Although telling the diagnosis is not usually a one-time affair, many parents recall a particular moment in time when the diagnosis, using the words HIV or AIDS, was first disclosed to their child. Some of their stories are told in the following chapter.

Chapter Summary

Secrecy Phase

Parent or family member learns diagnosis for the first time

- they are in a state of shock
- they vow not to disclose diagnosis to anyone
- they experience profound feelings of loneliness and isolation while outwardly attempting to project "normal" demeanor
- they need reassurance that confidentiality will be maintained
- they may identify one or more trusted adults with whom to share the diagnosis
- professionals at the hospital/clinic may be only people with whom parent can freely share feelings
- professionals should anticipate and meet parent's need for constant reassurance regarding confidentiality

Exploratory Phase

Parent or family member still keep the secret from most adults, but especially from children

- intensity with which secrecy is guarded is less marked
- they may show interest in meeting other parents in same situation, especially in parent support groups

- they recognize that support group members have mutual concerns about maintaining confidentiality
- they may display some ambivalence about keeping secret from child
- they may use support group to begin exploring feelings about disclosure to child
- they want to talk to child about clinic visits and treatment
- parent may join with professional in therapeutic play with child, especially over stress of treatment

Readiness Phase

Parent or family member moves closer to disclosing diagnosis to child

- they begin to activate plans for disclosure
- they may seek increased opportunities to collaborate with professional in planning for disclosure
- communication between parent and professional increases as they plan information to be given to child
- mutual respect for knowledge and skills of both parties highly in evidence in parent/professional relationship
- parent discusses possible "how to's" of disclosure with other parents in group, or with other trusted adult
- parent expands circle of adults to whom diagnosis is revealed

Disclosure Phase

Parent or family member discloses the diagnosis

- disclosure may follow a specific plan, in presence of, or in collaboration with, a professional
- disclosure may occur following child's direct questions
- disclosure may occur when parent feels an opportune moment has arrived, without professional presence or input

"Grandma, do I have the Eggs virus?" Kiyah asked.

CHAPTER V

Disclosing the Diagnosis

Disclosure of the diagnosis to infected or affected children is generally not a single act. More typically, the child learns the diagnosis over a period of time in the context of everyday life. However, there are times when a parent decides to formally discuss the diagnosis, either in response to the child's questions, or because she feels the time is right. Following are vignettes about disclosing the diagnosis. These stories illustrate the many ways that families have gone about sharing the diagnosis with their children.

The Story of Missy

Diane is the 34-year-old mother of two children — Missy, 11, and Shanell, 3. Diane was infected through sexual contact with Shanell's father, Doug, now deceased. Shanell was perinatally infected, and Missy is not infected. Diane has known Shanell's diagnosis for five months and has not yet revealed it to Missy, but she feels she must because she is afraid Missy will discover the diagnosis accidentally. As she struggles with her ambivalence, which she discusses with the child's medical team, she is encouraged to bring Missy to one of Shanell's clinic visits as a way to begin including Missy in the process. Predictably, this opens up many questions for Missy as she observes her sister's treatment and helps comfort her when she is distressed.

Initially, she asks about Shanell's IV gamma globulin infusions. "What is that?" She is told the name of the treatment and its purpose, "to prevent infections." Diane reports that between visits Missy's questions increase, and Diane consults with the team to get ideas about how to respond to Missy, without saying HIV or AIDS. At different times, Diane uses the terms "infection" or "special virus" or "blood problem" in describing Shanell's condition to Missy. Missy asks if "Daddy Doug" had the same problem as Shanell, and she is told he did. After some time, Missy asks her mother, "Do you have it too?" to which her mother again says "yes." At this point, Diane tells the medical team she wants to tell Missy the diagnosis. She prefers that it be done at home and asks the social worker on the team to be present "to help me in case I get stuck." A home visit is scheduled. Missy is told ahead of time that her mother wants to talk to her about her own and Shanell's condition. She also tells her that "Miss Mary" (the social worker) will be present. During the home visit, Shanell visits her aunt to provide privacy.

The social worker arrives at Diane's soon after Missy comes home from school. Diane invites Missy to sit next to her on the bed, which doubles as a couch, and the social worker sits in a nearby chair.

Mother: "Do you remember why I wanted us to have this meeting today?"

Missy: "To talk about Shanell and you being sick."

Mother: "That's right Missy, but first I want to ask you if you have any ideas about what is wrong?"

Missy: "Well, I know it's some kind of virus. Daddy Doug had it, and you have it, and Shanell, but not me. I don't know what it is called though."

Mother: "It is something called HIV. Have you heard of that?"

Missy: "I think so. I'm not sure. What does it mean?"

Mother: "Well, some people call it the AIDS virus too."

Missy: (alarmed) "You all have AIDS?"

(Mother looks over at the social worker as if for help)

Social worker: "Missy, your mother is trying to explain to you that she and Shanell have a virus called HIV and this is the virus that many people call the AIDS virus. Have you heard of it?"

Missy: (crying) "Does this mean Mommy is going to die?"

Mother: (puts her arms around Missy) "Missy, everybody dies sometime or other, but I'm not saying that I am going to die anytime soon. Mommy just wants you to know what's happening because you're such a big girl, and I think you have a right to know."

Missy: (as sobbing subsides) "Will you get sicker?"

Mother: "I hope not Missy because I am doing everything I can to keep well and to keep Shanell well."

Missy then says she is very tired and asks to be allowed to take a nap.

Over the course of the next few days, Missy experiences many changes in mood. At times she suddenly bursts out crying, sometimes becoming quite hysterical. At other times she becomes very withdrawn, often going to sleep soon after she comes home from school. However, after a few days she begins to talk about her next greatest fear. She asks her mother, "What will happen to me if you die, Mommy?" Missy is assured that her mother has already thought of this. She tells Missy that two of her favorite aunts would like to care for her in the event of Diane's death. Missy will be allowed to choose the aunt she wants to live with, and, with all the wisdom of Solomon, she asks her mother if, during the summer months, she might spend a little time with each aunt to "see what will be best for me."

With Diane's help, Missy decides prior to her mother's death which aunt she will live with. Diane then obtains the services of an attorney to draw up legal documents so that, in the event of her death, Missy's "chosen" aunt will become her legal guardian. Later, Missy says during a therapy sessions, "I think Mommy will not worry about me so much when she goes to heaven now that she knows who will be taking care of me."

Discussion of the Story of Missy

In this story the parent has chosen the setting and the circumstances under which to reveal the diagnosis. She has asked for the help of a trusted professional to support her, anticipating it will be a difficult task. Missy's initial reaction is to link the diagnosis to death. Diane uses words to reassure Missy that the emphasis is on staying well, while using actions (her arms around the child) to provide comfort for her feelings. Missy then retreats to the safety of sleep to provide a "buffer," or period of time out, from facing this new information. There are many fluctuations in Missy's mood as she struggles to come to terms with the implications of what she has learned. As she processes these thoughts and feelings, she comes up with specific concerns, such as what will happen to her if her mother dies. Again, she is able to get reassurance from her mother that plans are being made, and she is invited into the decision-making process, which empowers her to cope with her fears. Finally, Missy indicates her acceptance of the realities of her life when she expresses relief that her mother will not have to worry.

This vignette is not the end of the story for Missy and her family. Missy will undoubtedly experience many more changes of mood and behavior as she alternately confronts and denies knowledge of the diagnosis. Also, as new developments occur within the family — if her mother or sister became seriously ill, for example — Missy will face new and renewed fears. She will continue to need help and support as she copes with these feelings.

The Story of Kiyah

In Chapter I, Eva, the maternal grandmother of Kiyah, discussed her reluctance to share the diagnosis with an old family friend. Kiyah was then 4 years old, and Eva felt she was too young to know the diagnosis. As Kiyah grew older, Eva gave a variety of explanations in response to Kiyah's questions about why she needed to go to the clinic. For example, "You have to go and get a check-up and get some medicine so you won't get sick" or "You have to go because you are sick." To this, Kiyah retorted, "I am not sick," and Eva responded, "I know you don't feel ill, but you are a very sick little girl. It is because you take the medicine that you don't feel sick; the medicine makes you feel better."

Although these responses satisfied Kiyah, Eva awaited the time, which she felt sure would come, when she would have to give Kiyah more detailed information about her diagnosis. That day came when Kiyah was 6 years old. As in the past, Kiyah's questions followed on the heels of a clinic visit. Eva describes what happened.

> *Eva:* "At home, I had a copy of the book *Jimmy and the Eggs Virus* and I had left it laying around the living room for some time. At first Kiyah paid no attention to it, and I thought she didn't even notice it. Suddenly she picked it up and brought it to me and asked me to read it to her. The book is a story about a little boy who overhears his parent saying that he has the 'Eggs' virus. Later he learns that what he really has is the AIDS virus. I read the book to her all the way through. After I had finished reading it I asked her, 'Do you understand what it is about?' She said, 'Yes, it's about a virus.' She appeared to lose interest and went off to play.

> "Two days later, it was time for another clinic appointment. Afterward we stopped to get hamburgers. She asked me to take her to the bathroom and when we were in there she suddenly asked, 'Grandma, do I have the Eggs virus?' I told her that she did, and then I did my best to explain it to her, including using the proper names. I also told her that she could not tell anyone else about it. I explained to her that some people are not very nice about this illness. She seemed to take it all in stride, as she had done with my answers to her other questions in the past.

> "When we got home, she approached her brother Jameel and whispered into his ear that she had the Eggs virus. Jameel hit the roof; he was so angry with me, saying, 'Why did you have to tell her? She might go and blab it to other people.' I then reminded Jameel of an exchange he and I had had when his mother was in the intensive care unit at the hospital. We had come from a visit to her and were in the elevator when Jameel asked me if his mother was going to die. I told him that she would probably die soon. I

pointed out to him that just as his mother, my daughter, had told him the truth (about her diagnosis), he had also been told the truth by me. I said to him 'You can always rely on the fact that there may be some things in life that I choose not to tell you, and I will let you know when that is the case. But you can also know that when you ask me something that is very important, you will get the truth from me. Do you expect me to be any different with Kiyah?'

"After this, he went upstairs, and I knew he did it in order to cool off and think over the situation. Later he came back and told me he was sorry he had exploded and that, although he didn't really agree with my telling Kiyah, he thought she deserved to have her questions answered truthfully.

"The next day Kiyah went to school and, as I later learned, took the school principal aside and told her she had the Eggs virus. The principal told her that she already knew. Kiyah wanted to know how since 'it's supposed to be a big secret.' The principal told her that she had been told by her grandmother. The principal reinforced to Kiyah the need to keep the information secret because of the reactions of other people."

Later the principal called Eva and told her what had happened. When Kiyah came home that day, Eva discussed the issue with her and once again explained that this information was private and just to be talked about in the home and with the principal.

To date, Eva reports that Kiyah has kept the information to herself, and only discusses it with her grandmother.

Discussion of the Story of Kiyah

In this example, the grandmother elected early on to respond to Kiyah's questions as they arose. Thus, disclosure of the diagnosis was led up to gradually. Kiyah's early questions reflected the fears and concerns of young children about the medical treatments and painful procedures they experience during clinic visits. Kiyah's early questions reflected her need for explanations about the *purpose* of her clinic visits — "to get a check-up and get medicine so you won't get sick." Her grandmother's responses were developmentally appropriate and Kiyah gained comfort and confidence that she could ask and have her questions answered. Further, the grandmother had developed a consistent style with Kiyah, and with her older brother, Jameel. She allowed the children to formulate their own questions based on individual needs and concerns. She then provided simple and honest answers while preserving the adult prerogative of deciding that "there may be some things I do not wish to tell you, but I will let you know."

The Story of Marianna

Gina, the mother of 9-year-old Marianna, made an appointment with the social worker to discuss Marianna's questions regarding her illness and treatment. Gina said she believed Marianna had some suspicions about her diagnosis, but she was still unsure about whether she was ready to reveal it. The social worker suggested that sessions with both Marianna and her mother be established, and that together Gina and the social worker might begin to explore Marianna's concerns.

Upon entering the play therapy room, Marianna immediately went to the easel and paint supplies and created a vivid landscape with brilliant sun and lush vegetation. She next painted a family portrait consisting of a mother and two children. When Gina pointed out to Marianna that she had not drawn herself into the family portrait, Marianna laughed and said "oops," but made no real effort to complete the family circle. At this point, Gina, in some distress, picked up the paintbrushes and added Marianna to the picture. The social worker suggested to Gina that she address Marianna about her concerns. Gina asked Marianna, "Why didn't you draw yourself too? Aren't you a member of this family?" Marianna at first said she had "just forgot," then said, "maybe I went away and got sick." Any further probing by her mother met with shrugs of the child's shoulders, and the session ended soon after.

By their next session, Gina reported that Marianna had begun to talk more openly about her illness and treatment, and that questions about why she came to the clinic and why she got sick so often were increasing. Gina, until then, had told Marianna that she had "a special illness that makes your body weak so it is not easy for you to fight germs."

Marianna began to reveal the many concerns she had about her illness through her drawings, and the social worker facilitated dialogue between mother and child. After many sessions, Gina decided that she wished for professional help in disclosing the diagnosis to Marianna. A meeting with the mother, the child, the social worker, and the child's doctor was arranged. On the appointed day, they met together in a small consultation room at the clinic.

Gina: "You know how Mommy always likes to tell you what is going to happen when you come to the clinic?"

Marianna: "Am I going to take a test? Will you help me to hold still?"

Doctor: "No test today. We want to talk to you about why you have to come to the clinic, but we think you already have some ideas. Do you?"

Marianna: "It's because my body needs to get stronger. It's not good at fighting germs."

Gina: "That's right, that's because you have a virus. It's called HIV. Do you know what it is?"

Marianna: "Is it about AIDS?"

(Gina appears to be very emotional and has difficulty responding. She looks to the child's doctor to give assistance.)

Doctor: "Yes, HIV is a virus and some people call it the AIDS virus. Did you already have some ideas about it?"

Marianna: "Yes. I heard Mommy talking on the phone about it. Mommy thought I was asleep."

Social worker: "You have been keeping this secret for some time then. Has it been worrying you?"

Marianna: "Well, sometimes. Does it mean I will have to go into the hospital and miss school?"

Gina: "Oh! I think we are going to help you to keep very healthy."

Doctor: "We hope you won't ever need to be in the hospital, but, if you do, we have a teacher here who could help you with your work; and also, there is a playroom where you can meet other children."

Marianna then asked if she could go and join some other children in the playroom who were working on crafts projects. She left the room, running back to kiss her mother lightly on the cheek.

Discussion of the Story of Marianna

In this example, the parent wonders if her child knows the diagnosis, but has been unable to decide to formally disclose. She seeks the help of a professional in an effort to determine what the child actually knows before reaching her decision. The mother had frequently engaged the child's medical team in helping her explain specific treatment protocols to her daughter, and has stated how much she values this collaboration. It is not surprising, therefore, that she uses the team in helping with the disclosure. It is apparent from the child's easy manner that she had suspected the diagnosis. Her calm acceptance of the news, however, does not mean she does not have strong feelings, or that she misses the implications of the potentially fatal nature of AIDS. This awareness is clearly revealed in her drawings, where she is missing from the family picture. Nevertheless, her more immediate concern is with the possibility of missing the school she loves so much, and the professional team is able to reassure her about this. Once again, the child abruptly ends her participation in the session, demonstrating her need to control the amount of information she can effectively handle in one sitting.

In the months that followed, Marianna eagerly participated in the weekly play-therapy sessions, always insisting that her mother come also. Occasionally, Marianna's two younger siblings joined the session. It was in these sessions that all three children began to communicate to their mother their awareness of *her* illness and their fears that she might die. This became the basis of future work between the mother and the social worker.

The Story of Dana and Her Children

Another parent who waited for an appropriate time to tell her children about her diagnosis was Dana, introduced in Chapter I. At the time Dana learned of her diagnosis her children had just returned from an extended summer visit with their grandmother. Upon their return, they had to face the fact that their father had abandoned the family home, and their mother had suffered a miscarriage. Although she wished to tell the children her diagnosis, she felt they needed to have time to settle down and readjust to their home before placing any more "tremendous burdens" on their shoulders. After the children had been home one year, Dana felt that time had arrived.

> *Dana:* "By the time Alicia was 12 and Omar was 11, I had been diagnosed for just over a year. We had all gone through a lot of changes that year. When they had come back home after their summer vacation to find all the changes, although they were very sad and depressed at times, the three of us became very close. There were a lot of tears, but also a lot of hugging and kissing and being glad that we had each other. After that time, it seemed like they got used to being home, and then I began to see all the problems for them readjusting to our family again. Things has been very different when they had been with their grandmother. It seems like they had lived very wild and free, doing whatever they wanted. I had to help them get used to a more stable day-to-day life. Eventually they settled down, and so did I. I became less anxious about dealing with them, and they were definitely more relaxed. Now we could get down to dealing with the more day-to-day issues.
>
> "I found my opportunity to start leading up to telling them my diagnosis through some things that were going on at school. Alicia was getting to be a teenager, and was definitely beginning to show an interest in boys. Also, she was going through a lot of typical teenage stuff with girlfriends — one day friends with this one and one day

not. I noticed that one of the things that concerned her most about girlfriends was whether or not she felt she could trust them. It was clear that, to her, a 'good' girlfriend was one you could trust, one you could tell things to in confidence and 'know she won't go and tell the world.' Also, at this time, questions and discussions about sex and drugs came up a lot. Almost everyday, after they had done their homework and before they went to bed, we would end up in one of our little talks. It was after one of these times that I remember clearly thinking to myself 'now is the time to start leading up to telling them.'

"I felt that the very best way to try and get some points across to them and gain their trust was not to lecture them or give advice, but to talk to them about my own life, about choices I had made and decisions I had come to. I felt if I was very open with them, they would come to see that they could also be open with me about their lives, and see that they could tell me anything. So I began to tell them about the time in my life when I had started experimenting with alcohol and drugs. I had never used IV drugs, but I had used a lot of others. I told them how, at first I thought it would be fun, but later how many problems it had caused. I also told them that I was able to kick drugs because I was able to see, before it was too late, that I was not being a very good mother to them. I told them that they were babies at the time, and that even though I was using drugs often, I still loved them very much. I told them it was my love for them that made me able to stay off the drugs, and start being a better mother.

"They were totally fascinated by all this, I guess they had always thought I was perfect, other than yelling at them sometimes. I know they didn't think that I could understand about being tempted by drugs. The more I talked, the more they talked. They wanted to know more about my life, and they asked me why I felt their father had left. I explained that their father had not left because of them, but because he and I were having a lot of arguments. I told them we had argued because he wouldn't stop using drugs, including IV drugs. I also told them that I had discovered he had been unfaithful to me. Finally, I told them that I also discovered that I had become infected with the HIV virus through sex with him. This is how it went at that moment, and I remember it as clear as if it was yesterday."

Alicia: "What is that, HIV?"

Dana: "It is a virus, and it can lead to getting AIDS."

Omar: "It doesn't mean you are going to die, does it?"

Dana: "No. But it does mean I could get sick at any time if I don't take care of myself."

"At this point, I think it was such a relief to finally tell them, that I broke down and cried. Once I started crying, so did they, and we all started hugging and kissing each other, crying and comforting, all at the same time. When we all calmed down a bit, I explained to them that this is why I get tired a lot, especially after working all day. I guess I explained it in this way because I also wanted them to be more understanding and help *me* out more by doing their chores more willingly. I had found myself yelling at them a lot lately to get their chores done. I know that I was hoping that if they knew what was wrong with me, they would be more cooperative. I also hoped that this would create a lot of intimacy between us, and they would feel they could be open with me about their feelings and the things they faced with their friends. I wanted them to turn to me for information and advice, not feel they had to get it from friends who might advise them wrong. I also had to tell them about not telling others."

Dana: "Now I have told you all a lot of very private information, especially about HIV. I hope you realize that you cannot go about and be telling your friends and other people about all this. Some people are very ignorant about AIDS and also very foolish. They might try and do things to hurt our family if they knew. Also, because a lot of people are not very well educated about AIDS and HIV, they might think that you two have the virus, just because I have it. Then they might not want to be your friends."

"When I told the children about keeping it secret, I could see they really already understood this, so it wasn't hard to get it across. I did tell them which members of our family knew about my diagnosis, and so they knew they had other people than myself to talk to.

"Looking back on all of this now, I realize that actually *telling* them the diagnosis, was not nearly as difficult as having had to keep it a secret. Also, one thing that really surprised me was the way they reacted. I had expected them to be much more shocked when I told them what I had. I still don't know whether they were just pushing down their feelings about what I had. Another thought has since hit me about this — did they already have some suspicions about what I had? One thing I remembered looking back was that on the days I went to the clinic, even though I went when they were in school, it seemed to me on those days they always asked me how I was doing, and if I was all right. I wonder if I was somehow different on those days? I suppose I'll never really know."

Discussion of the Story of Dana and Her Children

In this example, Dana waited for two things to happen before she disclosed to her children. First, she waited until she felt the children were emotionally stable and ready to begin coping with the knowledge of her diagnosis. And second, she waited until an appropriate moment in time, when she could lead to disclosure by following up on some of the children's own questions.

Although some of the professionals Dana interacted with at the clinic had encouraged her to tell the children sooner, others had supported her decision to delay telling. Dana often said that although she looked to all of these professionals for support and information, ultimately, "I am the one who lives with the children every day of their lives, and nobody knows them as well as I do. It's good to get advice and ideas from the professionals, and the ones at my clinic are some of the kindest, smartest people I know. I trust them as much as some of my closest friends and family. But when it comes to my kids, I have to make the big decisions because I am the one who gets to live with the results of those decisions."

The Story of Amir

Amir is cared for by his father Raheed who is HIV infected but asymptomatic. Amir's older brother Khiree is 11 years old. All three family members arrive at the clinic, where Amir was tested several weeks earlier. The children are unaware that Amir has been tested for antibodies to the HIV. Raheed has requested that he be given the results of the test in private, without either boy present. Raheed expresses deep sadness, but little surprise, when he is told that Amir's test results show he is HIV positive. It was Amir's frequent upper-respiratory infections, as well as Amir's deceased mother's AIDS diagnosis, that led Raheed to suspect his younger son was infected. Soon after learning the test results, Raheed states that he wishes both boys to know the truth; however, he requests the assistance of the social worker in disclosing the diagnosis. A discussion then ensues between the social worker and Raheed about how best to approach the boys with this information.

> *Social worker:* "Have you thought about the possibility that the boys may have a lot of questions about AIDS? I wonder if you feel prepared to respond to the questions they may ask?"
>
> *Raheed:* "You mean about how Amir got it?"
>
> *Social worker:* "Yes, that is a strong possibility. I know your sons are very intelligent and tend to ask lots of questions. Also, they might ask about death, too. I wonder how far you would want to go in answering their questions, how you might want to handle it?"
>
> *Raheed:* "Wherever it has to go, that's how far. This is not a time for telling half the truth. Can't tell him he has the virus and then not tell him how."

Raheed asks that the social worker begin the dialogue because he fears that he will get "too messed up and say it wrong." Despite reassurance by the social worker that she would jump in and help if he had difficulty, Raheed prefers that she take the lead. Raheed agrees that he will join in answering any questions the children may have.

The children are then called into the consultation room by Raheed. Although the social worker had set up four chairs in a circle, when Raheed re-enters the room, he motions to chairs for the boys, and then pulls his own chair to the corner of the room, behind his sons' range of vision, but in direct eye contact with the social worker.

> *Social worker:* "Your father wanted you to join us here so we could all talk together about what he and I have been talking about. If you remember, last time you came, Amir had some blood taken for a test. The test was to tell us if Amir had a virus called HIV. Do you know what that is?"

> *Amir:* "Yes. That is the AIDS."

> *Social worker:* "Yes, you are right. HIV is not the same as AIDS, but some people call HIV the AIDS virus."

> (The two boys whisper together for a while.)

> *Khiree:* (pointing to Amir) "He wants to know if he is going to die."

> (The social worker pauses, and looks to Raheed to see if he intends to respond to the question. Raheed shakes his head and indicates that he wants her to respond. This interaction between Raheed and the social worker takes place repeatedly during the meeting.)

> *Social worker:* "Well, you know Amir, everything that lives must some day die. Every plant, every tree, every animal, and yes, every person will someday die. Everything that lives eventually dies. Most people die when they are older, but sometimes they die when they are young. I wonder if you asked this question because you have heard that a lot of people with AIDS die?"

> (Amir nods.)

> *Social worker:* "I thought maybe that was what you were thinking of. Maybe I should explain to you a little more. Right now you have something called HIV. That is a virus, and even though some people call it the AIDS virus, it is not the same thing as AIDS. It is true that some people with HIV do get sicker and then we call it AIDS. It is also true that there are a lot of people who have AIDS who die. But

right now you have HIV and you are just a little sick. That is why you have trouble with coughing sometimes."

Khiree: "That's why he gets the medicine, right?"

Social worker: "Yes Khiree, that's right. He gets medicine for his cough, and soon we will start to give Amir new medicine to help him to stay strong and healthy. Amir, I wonder if you know any things you can do to stay strong and healthy?"

Amir: "Eat the vegetables, they're good for you."

Social worker: "Yes, eating good, healthy food can help you stay healthy."

Amir: "No junk food?"

Social worker: "Well, maybe a few cookies once in a while, I know you guys wouldn't want to eat too much junk food."

(Both boys laugh. Then for a few moments, they engage in a lot of mutual teasing about who eats the most junk food. During this momentary respite, Raheed looks over to the social worker and smiles. Then the room becomes quiet again and Amir breaks the silence.)

Amir: "How did I get it, how did it get in me?"

(Once again there is nonverbal communication between the social worker and Raheed. It is clear that Raheed feels uncomfortable answering his son's questions, but he nods his head for the social worker to proceed.)

Social worker: "Amir, you became infected with HIV because your mother had it when you were inside her, before you were born."

Amir: "Well, how did she get it?"

Social worker: "She got it because your father has it. Do you understand how that could have happened?"

Amir: "When the mother and the father are in bed and have sex."

Social worker: "Yes, that is the way. I see you know a lot of things. Does someone teach you all these things?"

(Amir jerks his thumb behind him in the direction of his father.)

Amir: "He tells us all the things we have to know. But how did *he* get the virus?"

Social worker: "Well, your father has told me that he already told you he used to use drugs a long time ago. That was before he went into the prison where you used to visit him. He said he explained to you about drugs, so I want to know if you know something about drugs?"

Amir: "Yeah! That's about shooting up and needles and things."

Social worker: "Yes. Sometimes people use drugs that they put into a needle and then put it in their arm. I know your father told you he used to do that, but he doesn't do that anymore. Even so, sometimes people who use needles to put drugs in their body share the needle with someone else. Your father did this, and he probably shared a needle with someone else who had the HIV, and then when he used the same needle, he got the HIV in his body."

Amir: "Then my mother got it from my father. Did my mother know she got the AIDS when she had me?"

Social worker: "I don't think she did. Many times people do not know they have the virus because they don't feel sick. I wonder why you asked that question?"

Amir shrugs. He remains quiet for a while, then both boys ask if they can go and play in the playroom, and are given permission by their father. After the children leave, the social worker asks the father how he feels about the way the meeting went. He says he feels satisfied, but then apologizes to the social worker for not participating more. Raheed goes on to talk about the fact that he was incarcerated for over two years on a drug related charge, but feels he was more fortunate than most men because his sister, who cared for the children while he was away, brought the children to see him often. He explains that he used the very brief periods of time with them to educate them "especially about drugs" so that they would not get themselves into "the mess I put myself into." Raheed describes himself as a "street man" and a "man of plain words, street words." He says he does not "beat around the bush" when he is explaining things to his son, because "that is the way it is where we live." The social worker suggests that there will be a lot of opportunities to go over today's discussion with the boys, and then Raheed will be able to give the explanations the social worker has given in "the language the boys understand best."

At this point the boys return and Amir says he has another question.

Amir: "The people that do drugs, they bad, ain't they?"

Social worker: "Amir, I will answer that question in a minute, but first I have to ask you something. Have you ever done anything bad or that was wrong?"

Amir: (without hesitation) "Nope!"

Khiree: "Yes you did, yes you did. You stole my dollar from my piggy bank and then you lied and said you didn't do it, so that's two bad things!"

(Amir hangs his head in embarrassment.)

Social worker: "Did you do that, Amir?"

(Amir nods, still hanging his head.)

Social worker: "Then you must be a bad person, is that how it works?"

(Amir immediately jumps off his chair, and putting his hands on his hips, defiantly responds to the social worker.)

Amir: "I ain't bad, I ain't bad."

Social worker: "That's right Amir, and that is your answer. Sometimes people do something that is wrong, or maybe it is foolish. Sometimes people do things that hurt others, or hurt themselves. I think your father will tell you that doing drugs is not a good idea. It is against the law and it hurts your body too."

Raheed: "Haven't I always told you that. Anybody do drugs like I did is a fool. Then you might end up in prison like I did."

Social worker: "So Amir, now I have a question to ask you. Is your father bad?"

(Amir goes over to his father, holds his hand and leans against him affectionately.)

Amir: "My father ain't bad. He's good."

Social worker: "Well, I think you have the answer to your question about people who use drugs being bad. At some time we've all done something wrong or that we regret later."

Discussion of the Story of Amir

In this situation, the personal style and philosophy of the parent is very much in evidence. Raheed describes himself as a "street man" and a "man of plain words, street words," by which Raheed indicates that he prefers telling his sons the diagnosis immediately and directly. He appears to have no hesitation about disclosure, and in later discussions reveals he does not worry about the boys revealing the secret to others. He says that during the entire period of his incarceration, they did not tell their friends, so they are "used to keeping quiet about family business."

Despite the fact that Raheed's own style is usually very direct and graphic, when the meeting began he pulled his chair to the back of the room, and participated very little on the verbal level. However, through nonverbal cues, he directed the course of the dialogue. There was no doubt in the social worker's mind that if the dialogue had progressed along lines that were in conflict with Raheed's wishes, he would have interceded. As in previous examples, the boys took a needed "break" from the intensity of the experience when they acted playfully with each other and asked to be excused from the room. The fact that Amir's questions seem so direct and so controlled gives no indication of the actual intensity of feelings that existed in the room. In the discussion between Raheed and the social worker after the boys had left, Raheed confessed that despite his usual ability to approach the boys about difficult topics "head on," he suddenly "dried up" when the boys came into the room. He said "it was only then that I really began to think about how I could lose Amir." He also said that he wanted to see how the social worker would explain it to them. He said that although he had talked about drugs a lot to the boys, neither child had ever revealed their feelings about his past drug use, and that Amir's question about whether "people who used drugs are bad," had surprised him. He said it had been helpful to him as a father, to hear the way the social worker responded to that question.

From the vantage point of the social worker, the fact that these children had been told so much about their father's past life, and had often visited him in prison, meant that there were no difficult "family secrets" that had to be steered around. Although she would have preferred that Raheed do most of the talking, it was clear that he did not feel able. To insist on more verbal participation by him would have only made the experience more painful. As the parent, Raheed will be spending a great deal of time with his sons, and there will be many occasions for him to respond to his children's concerns.

Chapter Summary

The stories in this chapter depict a variety of situations. In some, only one family member is infected, in others, two or more members are. Some incidences of disclosure occurred as a result of a child's directly or indirectly expressed concerns and questions, while in others parents chose a particular time to disclose, sometimes with the help of a professional. There are probably as many different ways that children come to hear the diagnosis from their parents, as there are families affected; which is to say that there can never be a prescription for the act of disclosure.

It is important to remember that once the diagnosis is known by the child, the process is by no means over. Just as adults need repeated opportunities to talk about the diagnosis and its impact, so, too, will children. While many of the child's questions and concerns will be raised with the parent, or with the medical team, children can also benefit from a support group of their peers. These groups provide a forum for children to discuss the diagnosis, and work out their concerns and fears about the prognosis, treatment, and other related issues. Just as disclosure of the diagnosis is a gradual process, so, too, is learning to live it.

REFERENCES

Allport, G. W. (1958). *The nature of prejudice*. New York: Doubleday Anchor Books.

Boland, M., Tasker, M., Evans, P., & Keresztes, J. (1987, Winter). Helping children with AIDS: The role of the child welfare worker. *Public Welfare, 23*, 23-29.

Detwiler, D. A. (1981). The positive function of denial. *Journal of Pediatrics, 99*, 401-402.

Douard, J. W. (1990, Winter). AIDS, stigma, and privacy. *AIDS and Public Policy Journal, 5*(1), 37-41.

Goffman, E. (1963). *Stigma*. Englewood Cliffs, NJ: Prentice-Hall Inc.

Jackson, E. N. (1965). *Telling a child about death*. New York: Channel Press.

Keith-Lucas, A. (1972). *Giving and taking help*. Chapel Hill, NC: University of North Carolina Press.

Kellerman, J., Rigler, D., Siegel, S. E., & Katz, E. R. (1977). Disease related communication and depression in pediatric cancer patients. *Journal of Pediatric Psychology, 2*(2), 52-53.

Kubler-Ross, E. (1969). *On death and dying*. New York: MacMillan Publishing Company.

McFarland, R. (1989). *Coping with stigma*. New York: The Rosen Publishing Group.

Pearson, J. M. (1981). *Talking to terminally ill children about death.* Paper presented at the meeting of the American Academy of Child Psychiatry, Dallas, TX.

Spinetta, J. & Deasy-Spinetta, P. (1980). *Emotional aspects of life-threatening illness in children.* Rockville, MD: Cystic Fibrosis Foundation.

Waechter, E. H. (1971). Children's awareness of fatal illness. *American Journal of Nursing, 71,* 1168-1172.

CHILDREN'S RESOURCES

Aliki. (1987). *The two of them*. New York: William and Morrow and Company, Inc.

Baker, L. S. (1991). *You and HIV: A day at a time*. Philadelphia: W. B. Saunders Company.

Clifton, L. *Everett Anderson's goodbye*. New York: Henry Holt and Company.

Hausherr, R. (1989). *Children and the AIDS virus*. New York: Houghton Mifflin Company.

Hazen, B. S. (1985). *Why did Grandpa die?* New York: Golden Books.

Krementz, J. (1989). *How it feels to fight for your life*. Boston: Little Brown and Company.

Mayer, M. (1968). *There's a nightmare in my closet*. New York: Dial Books.

Merrifield, M. (1990). *Come sit by me*. Toronto: Women's Press.

Quackenbush, M., & Villareal, S. (1988). *Does AIDS hurt?* Santa Cruz, CA: Network Publications.

Rockwell, H. (1973). *My doctor*. New York: Harper and Row.

Rogers, F. (1986). *Going to the doctor's*. New York: G. P. Putnam's Sons.

Sims, A. M. (1986). *Am I still a sister?* Albuquerque: Big A & Company.

Tasker, M. (In press). *Jimmy and his family.* [Available May 1992 from the Association for the Care of Children's Health, 7910 Woodmont Avenue, Suite 300, Bethesda, MD 20814, (301) 654-6549.]

Tasker, M. (1988). *Jimmy and the eggs virus.* [Available from Children's Hospital AIDS Program, Children's Hospital of New Jersey, United Hospital Medical Center, 15 South 9th Street, Newark, NJ 07107, (201)268-8273.]

Viorst, J. (1971). *The tenth good thing about Barney.* New York: MacMillan Publishing Company.

Wilhelm, H. (1988). *I'll always love you.* New York: Crown Publishers.